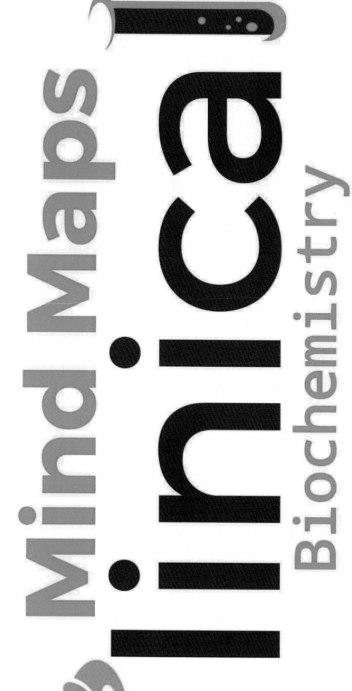

Mind Maps

Clinical

Biochemistry

Mohamed J. Saadh

Hala M. Sbaih

To order additional copies of this book, contact:
Xlibris
0800-056-3182
www.xlibrispublishing.co.uk
Orders@ Xlibrispublishing.co.uk

ABOUT AUTHORS

Mohamed J. Saadh, BSc. MSc. phD Biochemistry

Assistant Professor of Biochemistry, Faculty of Pharmacy, Philadelphia University, Jordan

P.O. Box. Philadelphia University-19392 Jordan

Mobile: +962 78 6945883

Email: mjsaadh@yahoo.com

Hala M. Sbaih

5th year student at the Faculty of Pharmacy, Philadelphia University, Jordan

P.O. Box: Philadelphia University-19392 Jordan

Mobile: +962 796811942

Email: hala_isbahe@yahoo.com

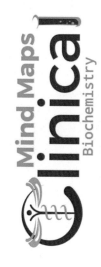

Mind Maps
Clinical
Biochemistry

TABLE OF CONTENTS

Mind Maps
Clinical
Biochemistry

Preface of the first edition

The purposes of the first edition is producing the first book of mind maps in clinical biochemistry that covered the fundamentals of Clinical Biochemistry to gain a clear understanding , providing detailed, specific information on the principles of clinical chemistry in laboratory diagnosis as well as the physiological changes that occur in disease and affect testing outcomes. This book aims to address new change in a variety of biochemical disturbance using diagramming tools, to generate, visualize structure, and classify ideas, and as an aid studying and organizing information, solving problems, making decisions and writing.

We continue to welcome constructive comments from all students who use our book as part of their studies and academics who adopt the book to complement their teaching.

Mohamed J. Saadh

Hala M. Sbaih

2018

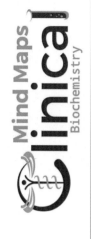

ACKNOWLEDGMENTS

At the beginning, thanks to Allah who gave me the chances to live and learn for everything done to me and for giving me more and more than I deserve. Thanks for your endless kindness and your generous courtesy and please accept this work.

Gratefully, I would like to thank the author Hala M. Sbaih, Pharmacist, Philadelphia University-Jordan for not only suggesting the idea for this book, but also for her invaluable assistance, comments, and continuous kind cooperation.

Finally, I wish to express our gratitude to all my colleagues at Philadelphia University-Jordan who have been supportive in the production of this new first edition, especially, Prof. Abdul Muttaleb Yousef Jaber, Dean of Faculty of Pharmacy for their kind help.

Mohamed J. Saadh

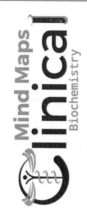

Mind Maps
Clinical
Biochemistry

Biochemical investigations in clinical medicine

you will organize your knowledge about :

The definition and importance of clinical chemistry

The types and uses of biochemical investigations

The specimen collection

The sampling errors

The urgent and repeated requests

The point of care testing

The precision and accuracy

The sensitivity and specificity

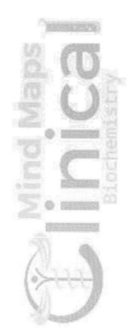

Mind Maps
Clinical
Biochemistry

9

Biochemical investigations in clinical medicine

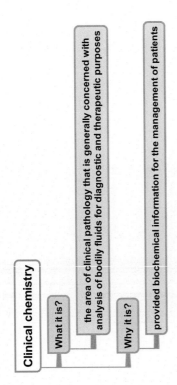

Clinical chemistry

What it is?
→ the area of clinical pathology that is generally concerned with analysis of bodily fluids for diagnostic and therapeutic purposes

Why it is?
→ provided biochemical information for the management of patients

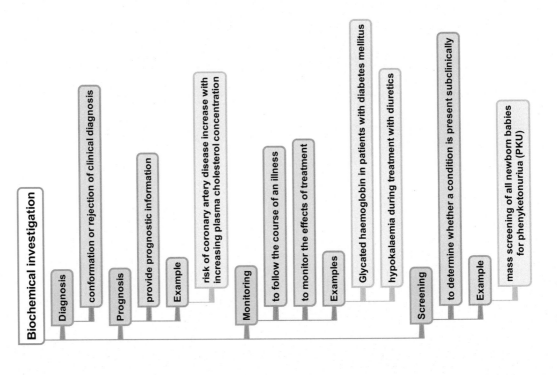

Biochemical investigation

Diagnosis
→ conformation or rejection of clinical diagnosis

Prognosis
→ provide prognostic information
→ Example
→ risk of coronary artery disease increase with increasing plasma cholesterol concentration

Monitoring
→ to follow the course of an illness
→ to monitor the effects of treatment
→ Examples
→ Glycated haemoglobin in patients with diabetes mellitus
→ hypokalaemia during treatment with diuretics

Screening
→ to determine whether a condition is present subclinically
→ Example
→ mass screening of all newborn babies for phenyketonuriua (PKU)

Biochemical investigations in clinical medicine

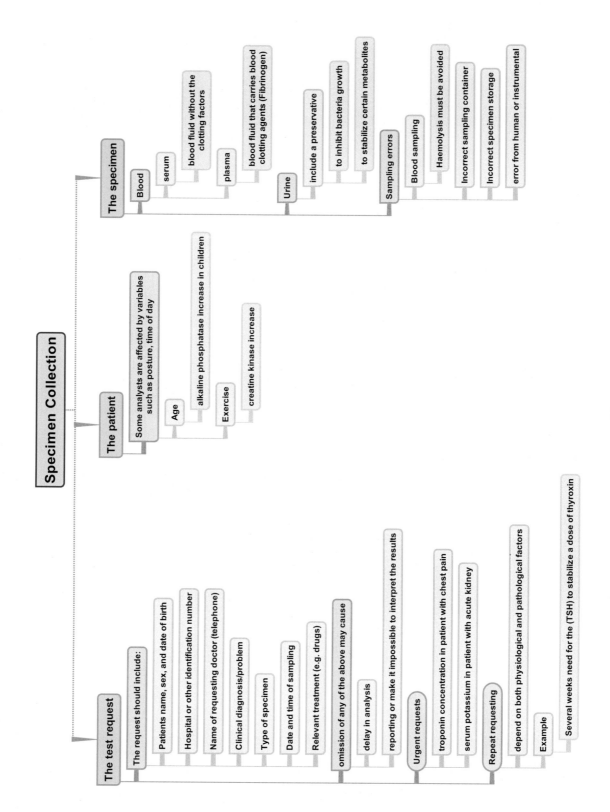

Specimen Collection

The test request
- The request should include:
  - Patients name, sex, and date of birth
  - Hospital or other identification number
  - Name of requesting doctor (telephone)
  - Clinical diagnosis/problem
  - Type of specimen
  - Date and time of sampling
  - Relevant treatment (e.g. drugs)
  - omission of any of the above may cause
    - delay in analysis
    - reporting or make it impossible to interpret the results
  - Urgent requests
    - troponin concentration in patient with chest pain
    - serum potassium in patient with acute kidney
  - Repeat requesting
    - depend on both physiological and pathological factors
    - Example
      - Several weeks need for the (TSH) to stabilize a dose of thyroxin

The patient
- Some analysts are affected by variables such as posture, time of day
  - Age
    - alkaline phosphatase increase in children
  - Exercise
    - creatine kinase increase

The specimen
- Blood
  - serum
    - blood fluid without the clotting factors
  - plasma
    - blood fluid that carries blood clotting agents (Fibrinogen)
- Urine
  - include a preservative
    - to inhibit bacteria growth
    - to stabilize certain metabolites
- Sampling errors
  - Blood sampling
  - Haemolysis must be avoided
  - Incorrect sampling container
  - Incorrect specimen storage
  - error from human or instrumental

11

Biochemical investigations in clinical medicine

Blood specimen tubes for specific biochemical tests.

Tube Type & Order	Common Tests
Sodium Citrate (BLUE)	**Haematology** : Prothrombin times, Coagulation Studies, INR, Factor VIII, Lupus Anticoagulant, D-Dimer, Protein C+S, APC, AT3, PFA100 (Platelet Function Test)
SST (GOLD)	**Biochemistry** : Lipids, LFT's U/E, Creatinine, SUA, Cardiac Enzymes. **Serology/Immunology**: Hepatitis A, B, C, Allergy, Rubella.
Plain (RED)	**Blood Bank** : Group and Hold, Cross Match **Biochemistry** : Therapeutic Drugs and Antibiotics, Serum Copper
ACD (YELLOW)	**Special Test:** HLA Tissue Typing, Flow Cytometry, (Lymphocyte Surface Markers, T&B Cells), HLAB27.
EDTA (PURPLE)	**Haematology** : FBC, Blood Film, Hb, WCC, Diff, Platelets, Glycated Hb (HbA1C) **Biochemistry** : Red cell Folate, Carboxy-Hb, Manganese, Ammonia, Homocysteine
Lithium Heparin (GREEN)	**Cytogenetics, Biochemistry** : Cholinesterase, Red cell &Insecticide - Organochlorines
Fluoride Oxalate (GREY)	**Biochemistry** : Glucose, Alcohol, Lactate
ESR (BLACK)	**Haematology**: ESR (Regional labs only)

12

Biochemical investigations in clinical medicine

Variation in results
- Analytical variation
  - Collected wrong specimen
  - mislabeling
  - incorrect preservation
  - Incorrect recorded
  - error from human or instrumental
- Biological variation
  - Actual changes in patients body fluids

Point of care testing

Biological compounds in blood and urine can be made away from laboratory by patients

- Advantages
  - immediate
  - quick
- Example
  - blood glucose

Category the tests can be made away from laboratory

- Test performed in medical to:
  - reassure the patient
  - further investigations
  - treatment
- Test performed in the home:
  - to give valuable information
  - (ex; glucose)
- Alcohol tests:
  - to assess fitness to drive

13

Biochemical investigations in clinical medicine

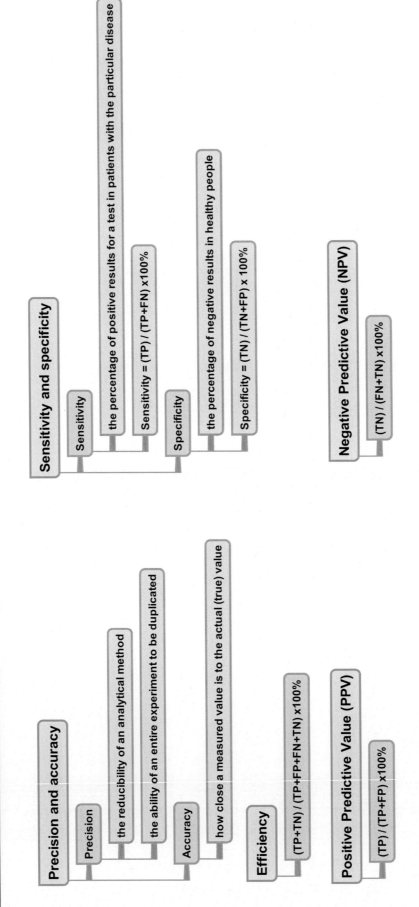

Precision and accuracy

Precision — the reducibility of an analytical method — the ability of an entire experiment to be duplicated

Accuracy — how close a measured value is to the actual (true) value

Efficiency — (TP+TN) / (TP+FP+FN+TN) x100%

Positive Predictive Value (PPV) — (TP) / (TP+FP) x100%

Sensitivity and specificity

Sensitivity — the percentage of positive results for a test in patients with the particular disease — Sensitivity = (TP) / (TP+FN) x100%

Specificity — the percentage of negative results in healthy people — Specificity = (TN) / (TN+FP) x 100%

Negative Predictive Value (NPV) — (TN) / (FN+TN) x100%

14

Precision and accuracy

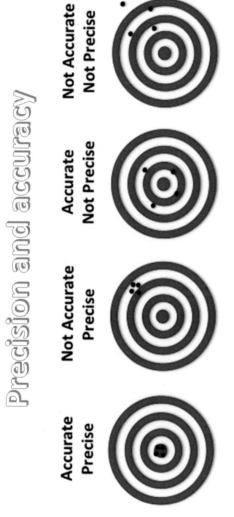

Accurate
Precise

Not Accurate
Precise

Accurate
Not Precise

Not Accurate
Not Precise

Sensitivity and specificity

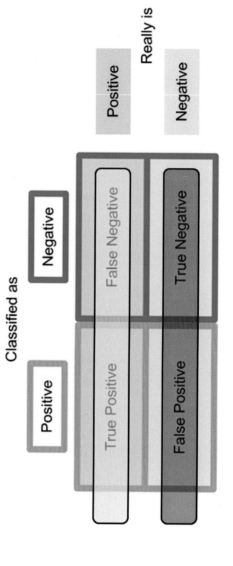

Classified as

Positive

Negative

Really is

Positive

Negative

True Positive

False Positive

False Negative

True Negative

15

Plasma proteins and enzymes

you will organize your knowledge about :

The functions of plasma proteins

The types of plasma proteins and their clinical significance

The types of plasma enzymes and their clinical significance

The enzymatic clinical diagnosis

The disadvantages of enzymatic assays

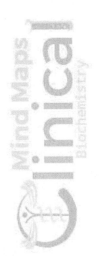

Mind Maps
Clinical
Biochemistry

16

Plasma proteins and enzymes

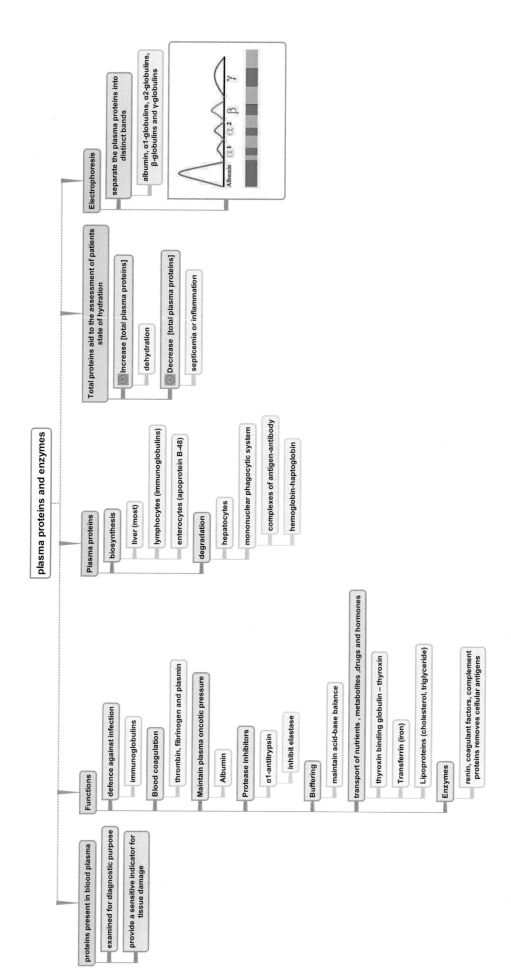

proteins present in blood plasma
- examined for diagnostic purpose
- provide a sensitive indicator for tissue damage

plasma proteins and enzymes

Functions
- defence against infection
  - immunoglobulins
- Blood coagulation
  - thrombin, fibrinogen and plasmin
- Maintain plasma oncotic pressure
  - Albumin
- Protease inhibitors
  - α1-antitrypsin
  - inhibit elastase
- Buffering
  - maintain acid-base balance
- transport of nutrients , metabolites ,drugs and hormones
  - thyroxin binding globulin – thyroxin
  - Transferrin (iron)
  - Lipoproteins (cholesterol, triglyceride)
- Enzymes
  - renin, coagulant factors, complement proteins removes cellular antigens

Plasma proteins
- biosynthesis
  - liver (most)
  - lymphocytes (immunoglobulins)
  - enterocytes (apoprotein B-48)
- degradation
  - hepatocytes
  - mononuclear phagocytic system
  - complexes of antigen-antibody
  - hemoglobin-haptoglobin

Total proteins aid to the assessment of patients state of hydration
- Increase [total plasma proteins]
  - dehydration
- Decrease [total plasma proteins]
  - septicemia or inflammation

Electrophoresis
- separate the plasma proteins into distinct bands
  - albumin, α1-globulins, α2-globulins, β-globulins and γ-globulins

Albumin α1 α2 β γ

17

Plasma proteins and enzymes

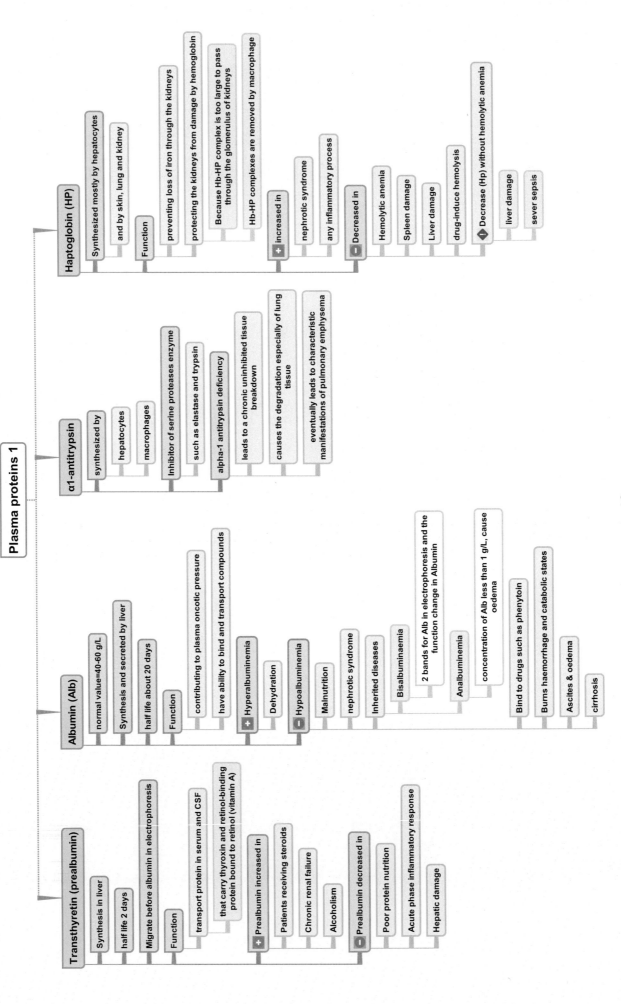

Plasma proteins 1

Transthyretin (prealbumin)
- Synthesis in liver
- half life 2 days
- Migrate before albumin in electrophoresis
- Function
  - transport protein in serum and CSF
  - that carry thyroxin and retinol-binding protein bound to retinol (vitamin A)
- **+** Prealbumin increased in
  - Patients receiving steroids
  - Chronic renal failure
  - Alcoholism
- **−** Prealbumin decreased in
  - Poor protein nutrition
  - Acute phase inflammatory response
  - Hepatic damage

Albumin (Alb)
- normal value=40-60 g/L
- Synthesis and secreted by liver
- half life about 20 days
- Function
  - contributing to plasma oncotic pressure
  - have ability to bind and transport compounds
- **+** Hyperalbuminemia
  - Dehydration
- **−** Hypoalbuminemia
  - Malnutrition
  - nephrotic syndrome
  - Inherited diseases
  - Bisalbuminaemia
    - 2 bands for Alb in electrophoresis and the function change in Albumin
  - Analbuminemia
    - concentration of Alb less than 1 g/L, cause oedema
  - Bind to drugs such as phenytoin
  - Burns haemorrhage and catabolic states
  - Ascites & oedema
  - cirrhosis

α1-antitrypsin
- synthesized by
  - hepatocytes
  - macrophages
- Inhibitor of serine proteases enzyme
  - such as elastase and trypsin
- alpha-1 antitrypsin deficiency
  - leads to a chronic uninhibited tissue breakdown
  - causes the degradation especially of lung tissue
  - eventually leads to characteristic manifestations of pulmonary emphysema

Haptoglobin (HP)
- Synthesized mostly by hepatocytes
- and by skin, lung and kidney
- Function
  - preventing loss of iron through the kidneys
  - protecting the kidneys from damage by hemoglobin
  - Because Hb-HP complex is too large to pass through the glomerulus of kidneys
  - Hb-HP complexes are removed by macrophage
- **+** increased in
  - nephrotic syndrome
  - any inflammatory process
- **−** Decreased in
  - Hemolytic anemia
  - Spleen damage
  - Liver damage
  - drug-induce hemolysis
  - **◆** Decrease (Hp) without hemolytic anemia
    - liver damage
    - sever sepsis

18

Plasma proteins and enzymes

Plasma proteins 2

α2-macroglobulin (α2M)

- Synthesis by
  - hepatocytes
  - macrophages
- Function
  - inhibitor of protease enzymes
- High M.Wt protein
- **+** increase in
  - nephrotic syndrome
  - large proteinuria
  - proteins are too large to be filtered though a damaged of glomerular basement membrane

Caeruloplasmin

- Synthesized in liver
- copper carrying protein in the blood
- functions
  - ferroxidase
  - superoxidase scavenger
- **+** increased in
  - Oestrogen-related effect
  - pregnancy
- **-** decreased in
  - Wilson disease
  - Nephrotic syndrome

Transferrin (TF)

- synthesize in the liver
- iron-transporting glycoproteins in the plasma
- control level of free iron in biological fluids
- Transferrin iron-binding capacity (TIBC)
  - medical laboratory test that measures the blood's capacity to bind iron with transferrin
- 2 mole of Fe+3 per mole of TF
- TF binds to Fe+3 transported by receptor-mediated endocytosis
- **+** increased in
  - Iron deficiency anemia
  - pregnancy
- **-** decreased in
  - Nephrosis
  - Liver disease
  - Hemochromatosis
  - Inherited disease cause accumulate of iron in tissue

Ferritin

- function
  - store iron in a non-toxic form
  - transport it to areas where it is required
- **+** increased in
  - hemochromatosis
  - Leukemia
- **-** decreased in
  - iron deficiency anemia

β2 microglobulin

- component of MHC class I molecules
- MHC1 present on all nucleated cells
- **+** increased in
  - multiple myeloma
  - lymphoma

19

Plasma proteins and enzymes

Plasma proteins 3

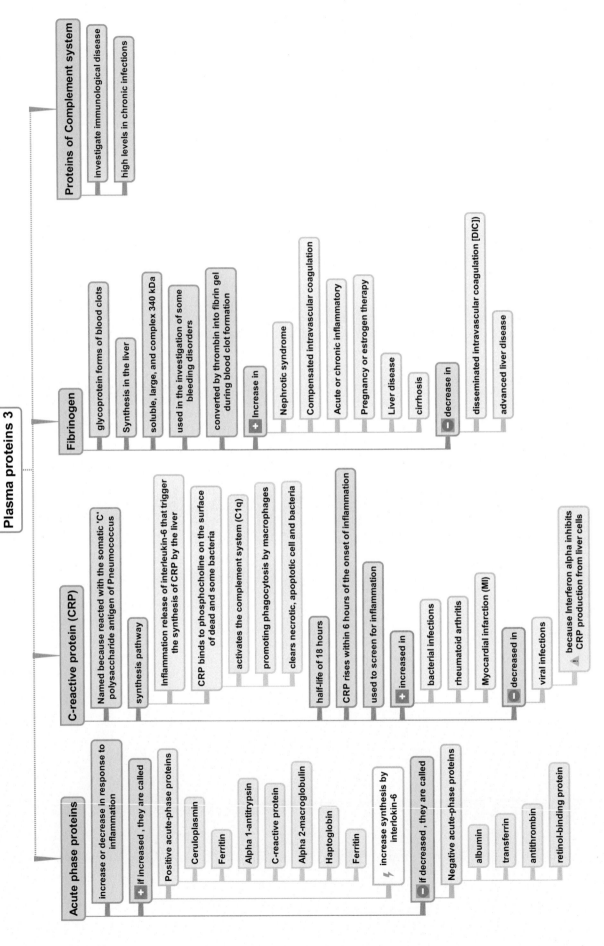

Proteins of Complement system
- investigate immunological disease
- high levels in chronic infections

Fibrinogen
- glycoprotein forms of blood clots
- Synthesis in the liver
- soluble, large, and complex 340 kDa
- used in the investigation of some bleeding disorders
- converted by thrombin into fibrin gel during blood clot formation
- [+] increase in
  - Nephrotic syndrome
  - Compensated intravascular coagulation
  - Acute or chronic inflammatory
  - Pregnancy or estrogen therapy
  - Liver disease
  - cirrhosis
- [-] decrease in
  - disseminated intravascular coagulation (DIC)
  - advanced liver disease

C-reactive protein (CRP)
- Named because reacted with the somatic 'C' polysaccharide antigen of Pneumococcus
- synthesis pathway
- Inflammation release of interleukin-6 that trigger the synthesis of CRP by the liver
- CRP binds to phosphocholine on the surface of dead and some bacteria
- activates the complement system (C1q)
- promoting phagocytosis by macrophages
- clears necrotic, apoptotic cell and bacteria
- half-life of 18 hours
- CRP rises within 6 hours of the onset of inflammation
- used to screen for inflammation
- [+] increased in
  - bacterial infections
  - rheumatoid arthritis
  - Myocardial infarction (MI)
- [-] decreased in
  - viral infections
  - ◄ because Interferon alpha inhibits CRP production from liver cells

Acute phase proteins
- increase or decrease in response to inflammation
- [+] if increased , they are called
- Positive acute-phase proteins
  - Ceruloplasmin
  - Ferritin
  - Alpha 1-antitrypsin
  - C-reactive protein
  - Alpha 2-macroglobulin
  - Haptoglobin
  - Ferritin
- ⚡ increase synthesis by interlokin-6
- [-] if decreased , they are called
- Negative acute-phase proteins
  - albumin
  - transferrin
  - antithrombin
  - retinol-binding protein

20

Plasma proteins and enzymes

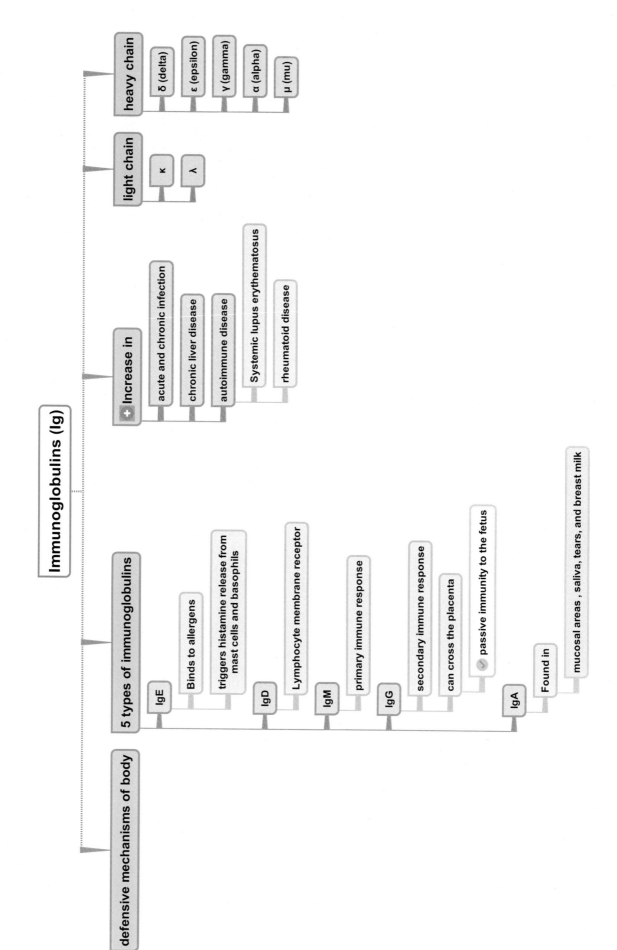

Immunoglobulins (Ig)

defensive mechanisms of body

5 types of immunoglobulins

IgE
- Binds to allergens
- triggers histamine release from mast cells and basophils

IgD
- Lymphocyte membrane receptor

IgM
- primary immune response

IgG
- secondary immune response
- can cross the placenta
- passive immunity to the fetus

IgA
- Found in
- mucosal areas , saliva, tears, and breast milk

Increase in
- acute and chronic infection
- chronic liver disease
- autoimmune disease
  - Systemic lupus erythematosus
  - rheumatoid disease

light chain
- κ
- λ

heavy chain
- δ (delta)
- ε (epsilon)
- γ (gamma)
- α (alpha)
- μ (mu)

21

Plasma proteins and enzymes

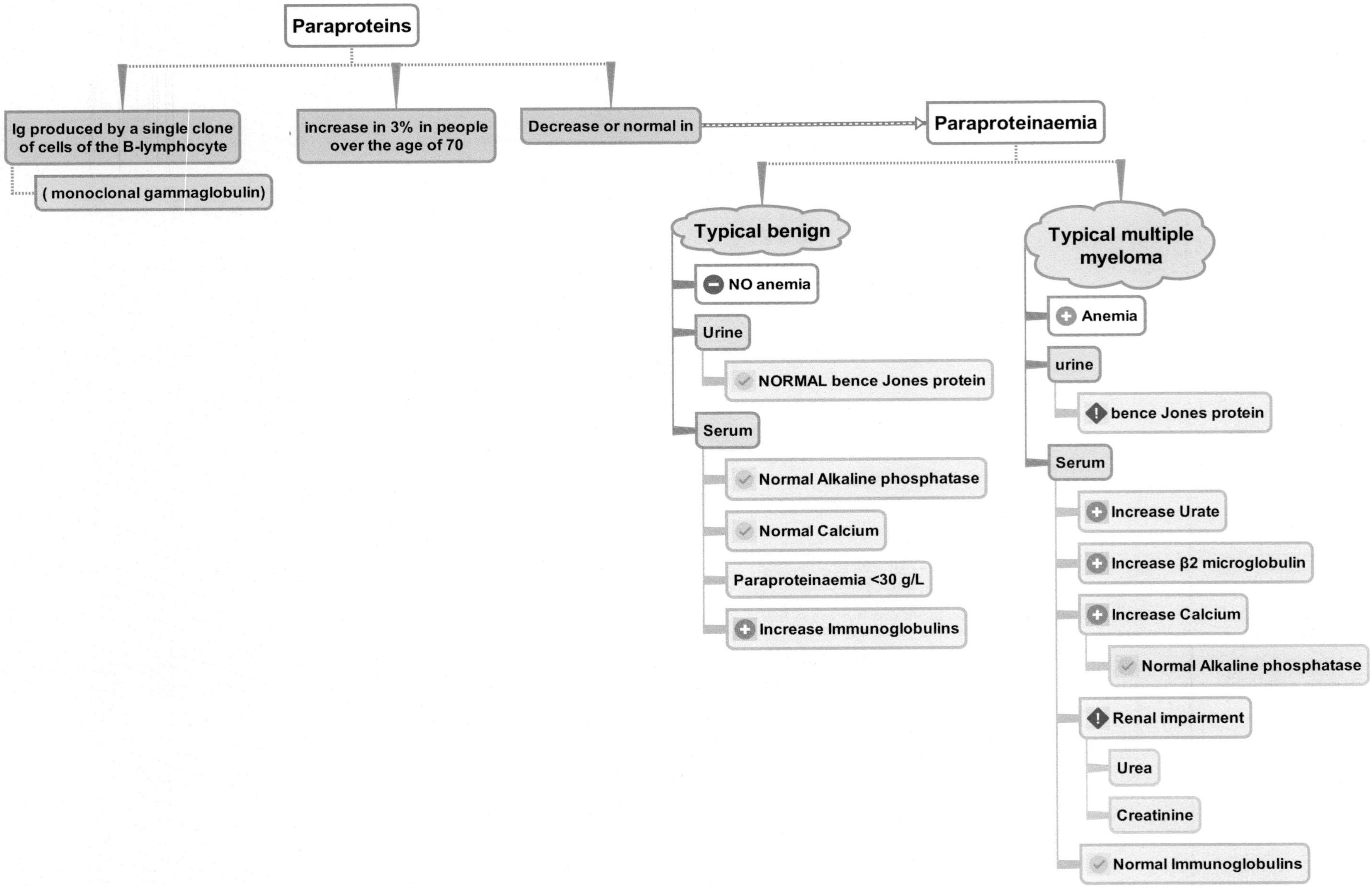

Paraproteins

- increase in 3% in people over the age of 70
- Ig produced by a single clone of cells of the B-lymphocyte (monoclonal gammaglobulin)

Decrease or normal in

→ **Paraproteinaemia**

Typical benign

- ⊖ NO anemia
- Urine
  - NORMAL bence Jones protein
- Serum
  - Normal Alkaline phosphatase
  - Normal Calcium
  - Paraproteinaemia <30 g/L
  - ⊕ Increase Immunoglobulins

Typical multiple myeloma

- ⊕ Anemia
- urine
  - ⬦ bence Jones protein
- Serum
  - ⊕ Increase Urate
  - ⊕ Increase β2 microglobulin
  - ⊕ Increase Calcium
  - Normal Alkaline phosphatase
  - ⬦ Renal impairment
    - Urea
    - Creatinine
  - Normal Immunoglobulins

22

Plasma proteins and enzymes

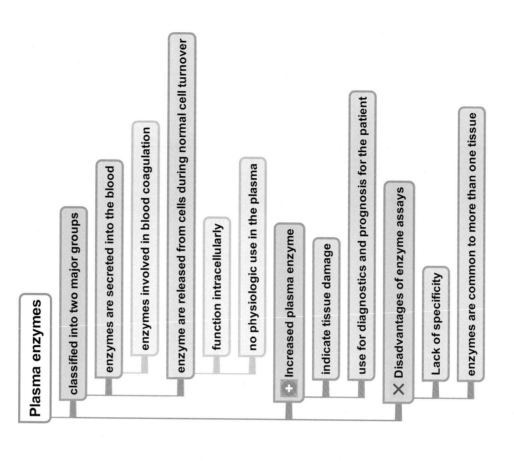

Plasma enzymes

- classified into two major groups
- enzymes are secreted into the blood
- enzymes involved in blood coagulation
- enzyme are released from cells during normal cell turnover
- function intracellularly
- no physiologic use in the plasma
- [+] Increased plasma enzyme
- indicate tissue damage
- use for diagnostics and prognosis for the patient
- [X] Disadvantages of enzyme assays
- Lack of specificity
- enzymes are common to more than one tissue

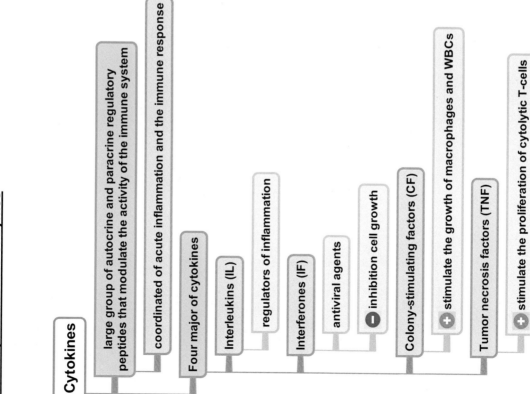

Cytokines

- large group of autocrine and paracrine regulatory peptides that modulate the activity of the immune system
- coordinated of acute inflammation and the immune response
- Four major of cytokines
- Interleukins (IL)
  - regulators of inflammation
- Interferones (IF)
  - antiviral agents
  - [I] inhibition cell growth
- Colony-stimulating factors (CF)
  - [+] stimulate the growth of macrophages and WBCs
- Tumor necrosis factors (TNF)
  - [+] stimulate the proliferation of cytolytic T-cells

23

Plasma proteins and enzymes

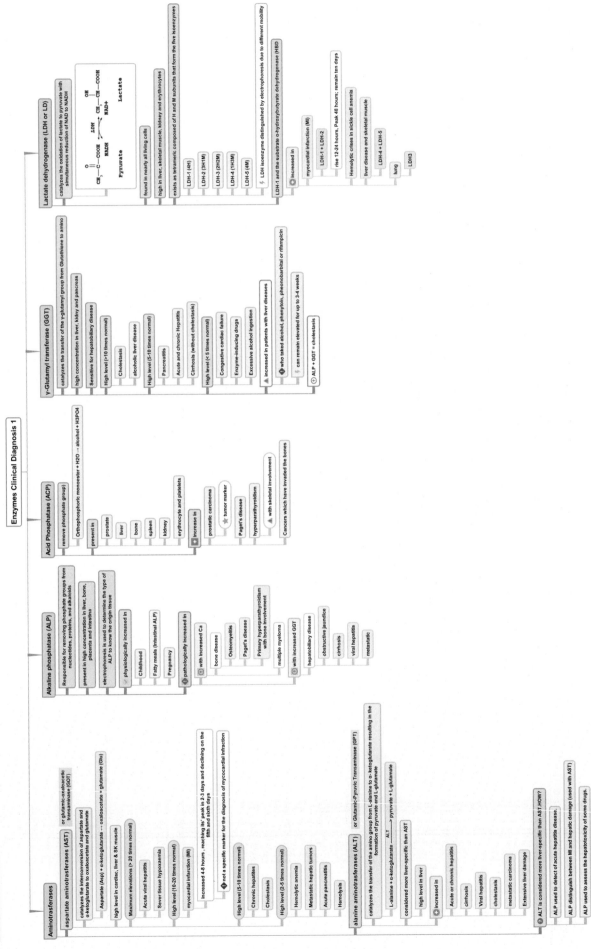

Enzymes Clinical Diagnosis 1

Aminotransferases

aspartate aminotrasferases (AST) — or glutamic-oxaloacetic transaminase (GOT)

- catalyzes the interconversion of aspartate and α-ketoglutarate to oxaloacetate and glutamate
  - Aspartate (Asp) + α-ketoglutarate → oxaloacetate + glutamate (Glu)
- high level in cardiac, liver & SK muscle
- Maximum elevations (> 20 times normal)
  - Acute viral hepatitis
  - Sever tissue hypoxaemia
- High level (10-20 times normal)
  - myocardial infarction (MI)
    - Increased 4-8 hours , reaching its' peak in 2-3 days and declining on the fifth and sixth days
    - ⊘ not a specific marker for the diagnosis of myocardial infraction
- High level (5-10 times normal)
  - Chronic hepatites
  - Cholestasis
- High level (2-5 times normal)
  - Hemolytic anemia
  - Metastatic hepatic tumors
  - Acute pancreatitis
  - Hemolysis

alanine aminotrasferases (ALT) — or Glutamic-Pyruvic Transaminase (GPT)

- catalyzes the transfer of the amino group from L-alanine to α-ketoglutarate resulting in the formation of pyruvate and L-glutamate
  - L-alanine + α-ketoglutarate —ALT→ pyruvate + L-glutamate
- considered more liver-specific than AST
- high level in liver
- ⊕ increased in
  - Acute or chronic hepatitis
  - cirrhosis
  - Viral hepatitis
  - cholestasis
  - metastatic carcinoma
  - Extensive liver damage

- ⊘ ALT is considered more liver-specific than AST. HOW?
- ALP used to detect of acute hepatitis disease.
- ALP distinguish between MI and hepatic damage (used with AST)
- ALP used to assess the hepatotoxicity of some drugs.

Alkaline phosphatase (ALP)

- Responsible for removing phosphate groups from nucleotides, proteins, and alkaloids
- present in high concentration in liver, bone, placenta and intestine
- electrophoresis is used to determine the type of ALP to know the origin tissue
- ☆ physiologically increased in
  - Childhood
  - Fatty meals (Intestinal ALP)
  - Pregnancy
- ⊕ pathologically increased in
  - ⊕ with increased Ca
    - bone disease
    - Osteomyelitis
    - Paget's disease
    - Primary hyperparathyroidism with bone involvement
    - multiple myeloma
  - ⊕ with increased GGT
    - hepatobiliary disease
    - obstructive jaundice
    - cirrhosis
    - viral hepatitis
    - metastatic

Acid Phosphatase (ACP)

- remove phosphate group
- Orthophosphoric monoester + H2O → alcohol + H3PO4
- present in
  - prostate
  - liver
  - bone
  - spleen
  - kidney
  - erythrocyte and platelets
- ⊕ increase in
  - prostatic carcinoma
    - ★ tumor marker
  - Paget's disease
  - hyperparathyroidism
  - ⚠ with skeletal involvement
  - Cancers which have invaded the bones

γ-Glutamyl transferase (GGT)

- catalyzes the transfer of the γ-glutamyl group from Glutathione to amino
- high concentration in liver, kidney and pancreas
- Sensitive for hepatobiliary disease
- High level (>10 times normal)
  - Cholestasis
  - alcoholic liver disease
- High level (5-10 times normal)
  - Pancreatitis
  - Acute and chronic Hepatitis
  - Cirrhosis (without cholestasis)
- High level (< 5 times normal)
  - Congestive cardiac failure
  - Enzyme-inducing drugs
  - Excessive alcohol ingestion
- ⚠ Increased in patients with liver diseases
- ⊘ who taked alcohol, phenytoin, pheonobarbital or rifampicin
- ↯ can remain elevated for up to 3-4 weeks
- ⊕ ALP + GGT = cholestasis

Lactate dehydrogenase (LDH or LD)

- catalyzes the oxidation of lactate to pyruvate with simultaneous reduction of NAD to NADH

$$CH_3-C-COOH \xrightarrow[NADH \quad NAD^+]{LDH} CH_3-CH-COOH$$

Pyruvate   Lactate

- found in nearly all living cells
- high in liver, skeletal muscle, kidney and erythrocytes
- exists as tetrameric composed of H and M subunits that form the five isoenzymes
  - LDH-1 (4H)
  - LDH-2 (3H1M)
  - LDH-3 (2H2M)
  - LDH-4 (1H3M)
  - LDH-5 (4M)
- ↯ LDH isoenzyme distinguished by electrophoresis due to different mobility
- LDH-1 and the substrate α-hydroxybutyrate dehydrogenase (HBD)
- ⊕ increased in
  - myocardial infarction (MI)
    - LDH-1 + LDH-2
    - rise 12-24 hours , Peak 48 hours; remain ten days
  - Hemolytic crises in sickle cell anemia
  - liver disease and skeletal muscle
    - LDH-4 + LDH-5
  - lung
    - LDH3

24

Plasma proteins and enzymes

Enzymes Clinical Diagnosis 2

Creatine kinase (CK)
- storage of energy in the form of phosphocreatine
- creatine + ATP ——CK—→ phosphocreatine + ADP
- exists as dimeric molecules composed of M and B subunits
- that form the isoenzymes
  - CK-MM
    - skeletal muscle
  - CK-MB
    - heart muscle
    - ⊕ CK-MB increased in
      - myocardial infarction (MI)
        - diagnosis by
          - CK and LDH isoenzymes
          - rise within 4–8 hours, and returns to baseline after 48–72 hours
  - CK-BB
    - brain
    - smooth muscle

Amylase
- found in
  - salivary glands
  - exocrine pancreas
- catalyses the hydrolysis of starch into sugars
- act on α-1,4-glycosidic bonds
- ⊙ Amylase increase in
  - acute pancreatitis
    - α-amylase starts to rise approximately 4 hours after the onset of pain
    - reaches a peak at 24 hours and remains elevated for 3–7 days
  - acute abdominal disorders
  - salivary gland disorders
  - macroamylasamia

Lipase
- catalyzes the hydrolysis of lipids to alcohol and fatty acids
- ◆ diagnosis & monitoring of
  - pancreatic diseases

Cholinesterase (CHE)
- secreted by the liver into the bloodstream
- break down an acetylcholine
- by preventing the accumulation of acetylcholine and the overstimulation of muscles and nerves
- symptoms of overstimulation of muscle and nerve fibers cause difficulty in breathing or death
- ⊙ Low plasma activity of CHE in
  - Liver disease
  - chronic hepatic dysfunction
  - pregnancy   Physiologically
  - medical applications
    - anaesthesia (suxamethonium)
    - Organophosphate (pesticides) poisoning
    - Cholinesterase test helps doctors determine whether or not an individual is poisoned

Alpha-feto protein (AFP)
- major plasma protein produced by the yolk sac and the liver during fetal development
- useful in monitoring the response to therapy of hepatocellular cancer
- ⊙ increased in
  - AFP levels (>500ng/ml)
    - >90% of patients with hepatocellular cancer
  - pregnancy   false positive

Troponin
- complex of three regulatory proteins (troponin C, troponin I, and troponin T)
- that is integral to muscle contraction, in skeletal muscle and cardiac muscle
- Specific to myocardial infarction
  - troponin T
  - troponin I
- Not specific to myocardial infarction
  - troponin C

25

The time sequence changes in plasma cardiac markers after acute Myocardial infarction

Cardiac marker	Start to rise (hour)	Time after infarction for peak rise (hour)	Duration of rise (days)
CK (Total) CK-MB	4-6	24-48	3-5
AST	6-8	24-48	4-6
LDH/HBD LDH₁ / LDH₂	12-24	48-72	7-12
Myoglobin	2-4	12-24	2-4
Troponin TnI, TnT	4-6	12-24	7-10
CRP	4-6	12-24	3-5

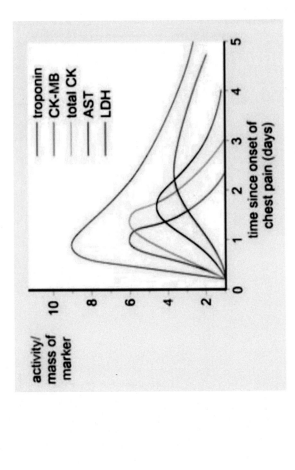

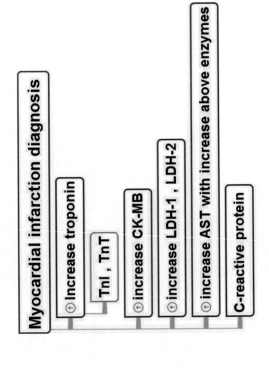

26

Plasma proteins and enzymes

Emphysema

- condition in which there is over-inflation of structures in the lungs known as alveoli
- The walls between the alveoli within the lungs lose their ability to stretch and recoil
- Lung elasticity is lost, which causes air to get trapped in the alveoli impairing the exchange of oxygen and carbon dioxide
- airflow obstruction occurs when the support of the airway is lost

Causes of Emphysema
- Cigarette smoking
- Deficiency of a "lung protector" protein known as alpha 1-antitrypsin

Symptoms of Emphysema
- Shortness of breath
- Coughing
- A limited exercise tolerance

Normal Alveoli

Emphysematous Alveoli

Treatment
- Quitting smoking is the single most important factor for maintaining healthy lungs
- Bronchodilator drugs prescribed by a doctor
- Antibiotics
- Exercise including breathing exercises
- Treatment with Alpha I-Proteinase Inhibitor for persons with AAT deficiency-related emphysema
- Lung transplant

Prevention
- Do not smoke
- Regular checkups with a doctor
- Maintain good health habits overall (proper nutrition, adequate rest, regular exercise)
- Reduce chances of possible exposure to air pollution

Plasma proteins and enzymes

Anemia

Aplastic Anemia

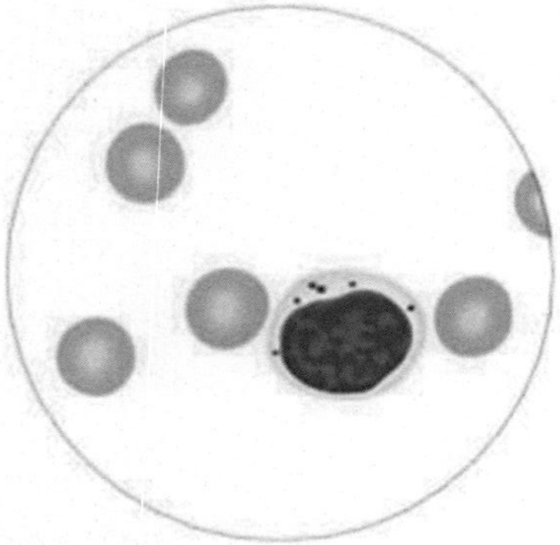

Normocytic, Normochromic Anemia Illustration of abnormal blood cells found under microscopic inspection of a blood sample with normocytic, normochromic anemia

Iron Deficiency Anemia

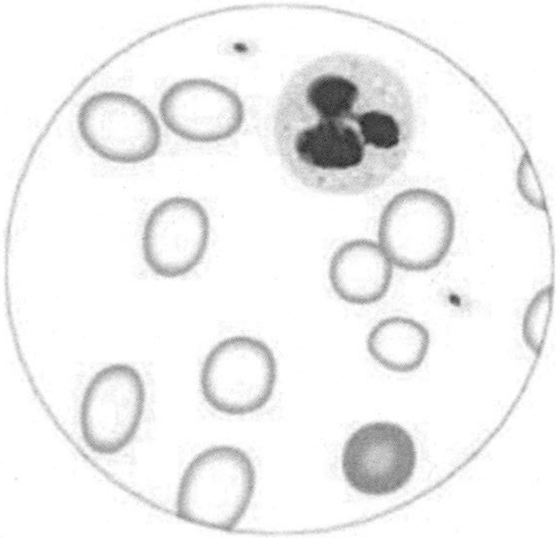

Microcytic, Hypochromic Anemia Illustration of abnormal blood cells found under microscopic inspection of a blood sample with iron deficiency anemia

Pernicious Anemia

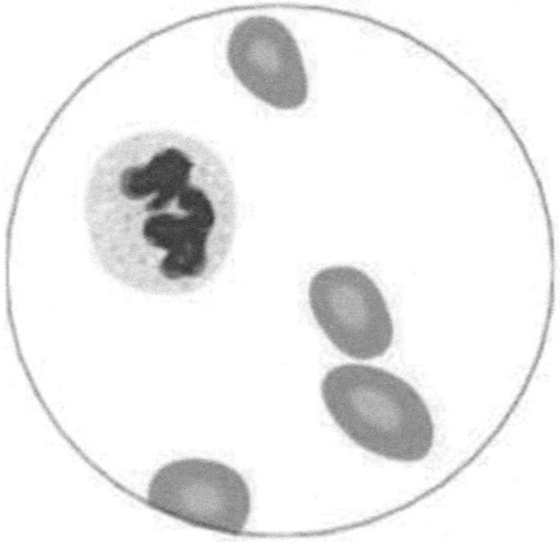

Macrocytic, Normochromic Anemia Illustration of abnormal blood cells found under microscopic inspection of a blood sample with pernicious anemia

Plasma proteins and enzymes

Pneumonia

Pneumonia is an infection in one or both of the lungs. Many small germs, such as bacteria, viruses, and fungi, can cause pneumonia

symptoms

- coughing that may produce phlegm (mucus)
- fever, sweating, and chills
- shortness of breath
- chest pain
- Symptoms by cause
  - Viral pneumonia may start with flu-like symptoms, such as wheezing. A high fever may occur after 12–36 hours
  - Bacterial pneumonia may cause a fever as high as 105°F along with profuse sweating, bluish lips and nails, and confusion.
- Symptoms by age
  - Children under 5 years of age may have fast breathing.
  - Infants may vomit, lack energy, or have trouble drinking or eating.
  - Older people may have a lower-than-normal body temperature.

types

- Types by germ
  - Bacterial pneumonia
  - Viral pneumonia
  - Mycoplasma pneumonia
  - Fungal pneumonia
- Types by location
  - Hospital-acquired pneumonia (HAP)
  - Community-acquired pneumonia (CAP)
- Types by how they are acquired
  - Aspiration pneumonia
  - Ventilator-associated pneumonia (VAP)

Diagnosis

- blood test
- sputum test
- Pulse oximetry
  - oxygen sensor placed on one of fingers can indicate whether lungs are moving enough oxygen through bloodstream
- urine test
- CT scan
- fluid sample
- bronchoscopy

treatment

- Home treatment
  - taking drugs as prescribed
  - getting a lot of rest
  - drinking plenty of fluids
  - not overdoing it by going back to school or work too soon
- Hospitalization
  - Intravenous antibiotics
  - Respiratory therapy
  - Oxygen therapy

prevention

- Pneumonia vaccine
  - Prevnar 13 — The Centers for Disease Control and Prevention (CDC) recommends this vaccine for:
    - babies and children under the age of 2
    - adults ages 65 years or older
    - people between ages 2 and 65 years with chronic conditions that increase their risk of pneumonia
  - Pneumovax 23 — The Centers for Disease Control and Prevention (CDC) recommends this vaccine for:
    - adults ages 65 years or older
    - adults ages 19–64 years who smoke
    - people between ages 2 and 65 years with chronic conditions that increase their risk of pneumonia
- If you smoke, try to quit. Smoking makes you more susceptible to respiratory infections, especially pneumonia
- Wash your hands regularly with soap and water.
- Cover your coughs and sneezes, and dispose of used tissues promptly.
- Maintain a healthy lifestyle to strengthen your immune system. Get enough rest, eat a healthy diet, and get regular exercise.

Lungs showing two types of pneumonia, (left) lobar and (right) lobular

Lobar
Lobular

Microscopic view shows bacteria responsible for fluid build-up

29

Plasma proteins and enzymes

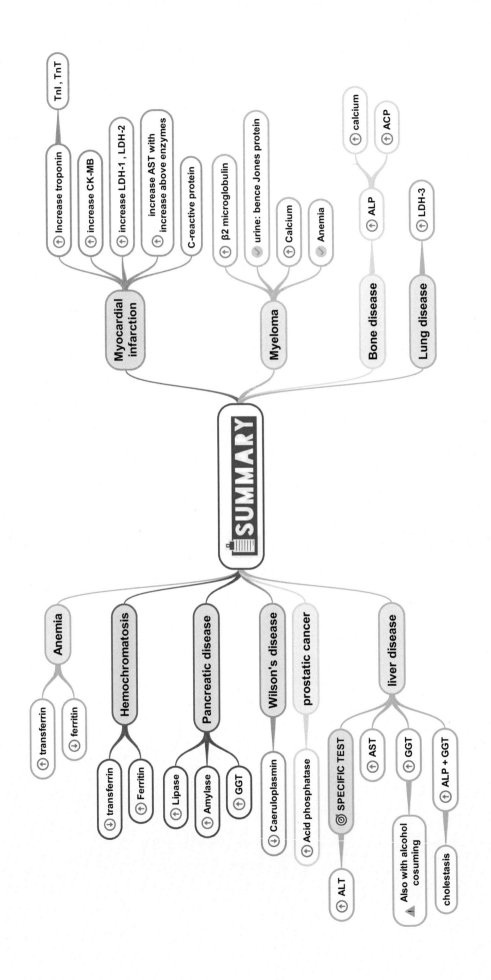

Plasma proteins and enzymes

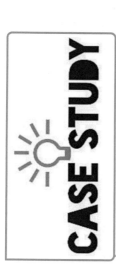

CASE STUDY

A 66-year-old male was sent by his GP to casualty because of tight chest pain that had occurred 3 days previously . The pain had largely resolved after 6 hours , but he was left feeling weak and breathless , which worsened over a few days , causing him eventually to seek medical attention.

The following laboratory test results were found

Plasma

Creatine kinase 235 U/L (<250)

Troponin T 0.13 µg/L (<0.1)

An ECG showed changes suggestive of a myocardial infarction in the lateral leads V4-V7

Discussion

The plasma CK activity has returned to normal , because of the time delay since myocardial infarction

Whilst the plasma troponin T concentration still remain elevated

Plasma CK usually starts to rise 4-6 hours after a myocardial infarction and to a normalize at about 3-5 days.

Plasma troponin T starts to rise at 4-6 hours post-infarct

remain elevated for as long as about 10 days

Troponins are useful cardiac markers in both the early hours and a few days later

The liver

you will organize your knowledge about :

- The physiology, structure and functions of liver
- The liver diseases, causes and clinical markers
- The liver function test (LFTs)
- The types of jaundice
- The use of GPT/GOT ratio in clinical diagnosis
- The fatty liver disease
- The progression of liver diseases

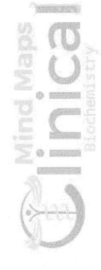

Mind Maps
Clinical
Biochemistry

32

The liver

The liver

- performs an astonishingly large number of tasks that impact all body systems
- the largest organ in the body
- vital importance in
  - intermediary metabolism
  - detoxification
  - elimination of toxic substance

Structure of liver

- 60% hepatocytes
- 30% kupffer cell (reticuloendothelial)
- 10% Supporting tissue

The anatomy of the liver at the cellular level

- have two channels that can supply and oxygen nutriment
  - hepatic artery
  - hepatic portal vein
- The corresponding channels is
  - hepatic vein and bile ducts

The liver

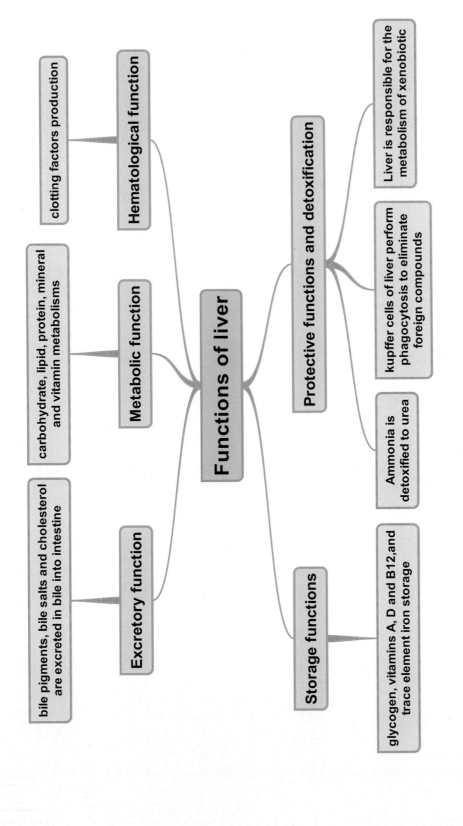

Functions of liver

- **Hematological function**
  - clotting factors production
- **Metabolic function**
  - carbohydrate, lipid, protein, mineral and vitamin metabolisms
- **Excretory function**
  - bile pigments, bile salts and cholesterol are excreted in bile into intestine
- **Protective functions and detoxification**
  - Liver is responsible for the metabolism of xenobiotic
  - kupffer cells of liver perform phagocytosis to eliminate foreign compounds
  - Ammonia is detoxified to urea
- **Storage functions**
  - glycogen, vitamins A, D and B12,and trace element iron storage

34

The liver

Liver function tests (LFTs)

groups of blood tests that give information about the state of a patient's liver and can contribute to making an accurate diagnosis of the specific liver disorder

comprises of
- Total protein
- Albumin and globulin
- Prothrombin Time
- Transaminases such as AST & ALT
- Alkaline phosphatase
- Bilirubin
- Gamma Glutamyl Transpeptidase (GGT)

LFTs are divided into
- true tests of liver function
  - serum albumin, bilirubin, and Prothrombin time
- tests that are indicators of liver injury or biliary tract disease

are often given in the following situations:
- to screen for liver infections, such as hepatitis C
- to monitor the side effects of certain medications known to affect the liver
- if you already have a liver disease, to monitor the disease and how well a particular treatment is working
- to measure the degree of scarring (cirrhosis) on the liver
- if you're experiencing the symptoms of a liver disorder
- if you're planning on becoming pregnant

How a liver function test is performed
1. The healthcare provider will clean your skin before the test to prevent any microorganisms on your skin from contaminating the test.
2. They'll likely wrap a cuff or some sort of pressure device on your arm. This will help your veins become more visible. They will use a needle to draw several samples of blood from your arm.
3. After the draw, the healthcare provider will place some gauze and a bandage over the puncture site. Then they will send the blood sample to a laboratory for testing.

The risks of a liver function test
- bleeding under the skin, or hematoma
- fainting
- infection

After a liver function test
After the test, you can usually leave and go about your life as usual. However, if you feel faint or lightheaded during the blood draw, you should rest before you leave the testing facility.

The liver

Liver diseases

Hemochromatosis

Hemochromatosis allows iron to deposit in the liver, damaging it

The iron also deposits throughout the body, causing multiple other health problems.

Primary biliary cirrhosis

In this rare disorder, an unclear process slowly destroys the bile ducts in the liver. Permanent liver scarring (cirrhosis) eventually develops

Cirrhosis

fibrosis, shrinkage liver, decrease number and function of hepatocellular

Jaundice

high plasma concentration of bilirubin

Cholestasis

decrease in bile flow due to impaired secretion by hepatocytes or to obstruction of bile flow through intra-or extrahepatic bile ducts

Liver cancer

occurs after cirrhosis is present

AFP

Hepatitis

acute or chronic damage to and destruction of liver

non-infectious causes

heavy drinking, drugs, allergic reactions, or obesity

Inflammation of the liver, usually caused by viruses like hepatitis A, B, and C

Ascites

As cirrhosis results, the liver leaks fluid (ascites) into the belly, which becomes distended and heavy

Primary sclerosing cholangitis

A rare disease with unknown causes, primary sclerosing cholangitis causes inflammation and scarring in the bile ducts in the liver

Liver failure

has many causes including infection, genetic diseases, and excessive alcohol

The liver

Detoxification
- urea

Excretion
- bile pigments, bile salts

Classification of liver functions test

Serum enzymes
- Transaminase (ALT, AST)
- alkaline phosphate (ALP)
  - ⊕ Increase (total bilirubin and ALP)
  - ⊕ OR (ALP and GGT)
  - ➢ cholestasis
  - Good indicator of intrahepatic disease due to extra-hepatic obstruction
- 5'-nucleotidase
  - cholestasis or damage to the intra- or extrahepatic biliary system
- LDH isoenzyme

Synthetic function
- Prothrombin time
  - Good indicator of intrahepatic disease due to extra-hepatic obstruction
- serum albumin

Metabolic capacity
- Galactose tolerance
- antipyrine clearance

urine/(faeces)

Urobilin
- Urobilin is the final product of oxidation of urobilinogen by oxygen by air
- The amount change with the amount of urobilinogen excretion

urobilinogen
- Conjugated bilirubin is excreted via bile salts to intestine
- Bacteria in the intestine break down bilirubin to urobilinogen for excretion in the feces
- normal value for fecal urobilinogen = 40 - 280 mg/day

Bilirubinurine

- Bilirubin is not normally present in urine and faese
  - since bacteria in intestine reduce it to urobilinogen
- kidneys do not filter unconjugated bilirubin because of its avid binding to albumin
  - bilirubin-albumin complex is too large
- conjugated bilirubin can pass through glomerular filter
- Bilirubin is found in the urine in obstructive jaundice due to various causes and in cholestasis
  - Bilirubin in the urine may be detected even before clinical jaundice is noted.
  - Bilirubin is used to diagnosis of jaundice

three major causes of increased serum bilirubin
- Hemolytic Jaundice
  - ⊕ total bilirubin
  - direct bilirubin (conjugated) is usually normal
  - Urine color is normal
  - ✗ no bilirubin found in urine
- Hepatic Jaundice
  - occur in viral hepatitis
  - ⊕ direct and indirect bilirubin
  - Urine color is dark
  - ➢ bilirubin is present in the urine
- Obstructive jaundice (Cholestasis)
  - ⊕ direct and indirect bilirubin
  - Urine color is dark
  - ➢ bilirubin is present in the urine

Abnormal bilirubin levels can be found in many disorders, including
- blocked bile ducts
- liver diseases
- Cirrhosis
- hepatitis
- immature liver development in newborns

The liver

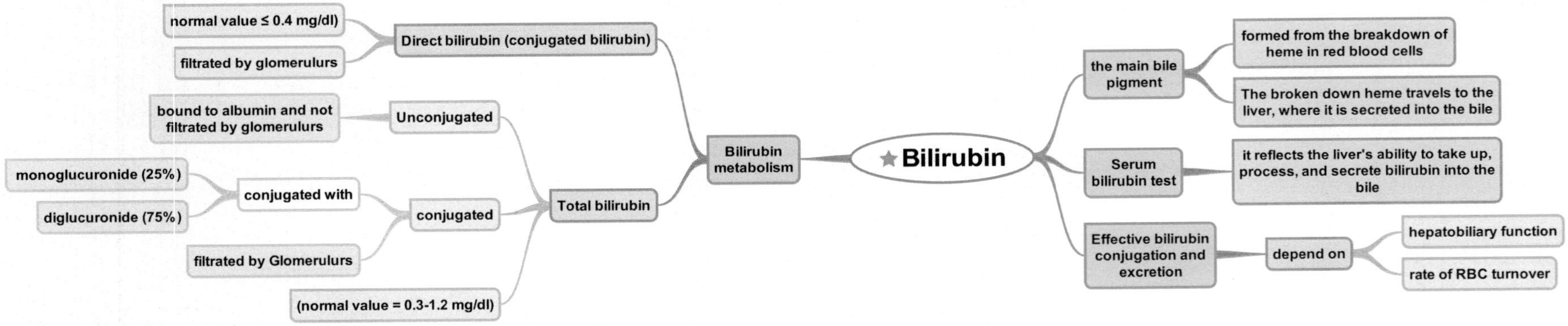

Bilirubin

- the main bile pigment
  - formed from the breakdown of heme in red blood cells
  - The broken down heme travels to the liver, where it is secreted into the bile

- Serum bilirubin test
  - it reflects the liver's ability to take up, process, and secrete bilirubin into the bile

- Effective bilirubin conjugation and excretion
  - depend on
    - hepatobiliary function
    - rate of RBC turnover

Bilirubin metabolism

- Direct bilirubin (conjugated bilirubin)
  - normal value ≤ 0.4 mg/dl
  - filtrated by glomerulurs

- Total bilirubin
  - Unconjugated
    - bound to albumin and not filtrated by glomerulurs
  - conjugated
    - conjugated with
      - monoglucuronide (25%)
      - diglucuronide (75%)
    - filtrated by Glomerulurs
  - (normal value = 0.3-1.2 mg/dl)

The liver

Bilirubin metabolism

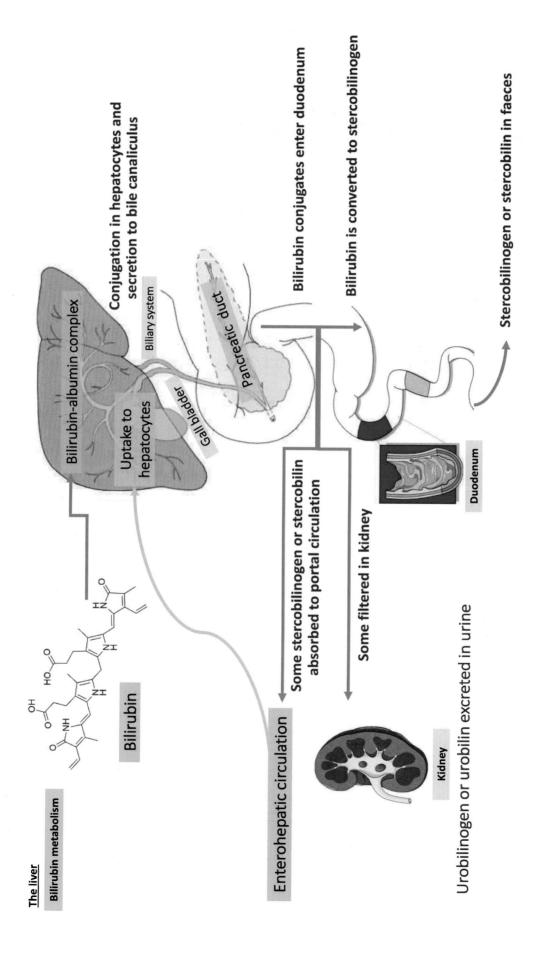

Bilirubin

Bilirubin-albumin complex

Uptake to hepatocytes

Conjugation in hepatocytes and secretion to bile canaliculus

Biliary system

Gall bladder

Pancreatic duct

Bilirubin conjugates enter duodenum

Bilirubin is converted to stercobilinogen

Stercobilinogen or stercobilin in faeces

Duodenum

Some stercobilinogen or stercobilin absorbed to portal circulation

Some filtered in kidney

Enterohepatic circulation

Kidney

Urobilinogen or urobilin excreted in urine

39

Differences of two Bilirubins

	Free Bilirubin	Conjugated Bilirubin
Binding with Glucuronic acid	No	yes
Reacting with diazo reagent	Slow & indirect	Rapid & direct
Solubility in water	Small	Large
Discharged via kidney	No	yes
Pass through the membrane of cell	yes	No

40

The liver

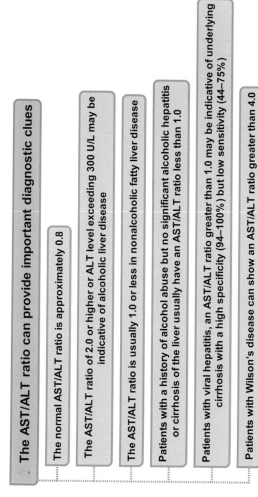

GPT/GOT ratio

AST=GOT
ALT=GPT

normal

GPT/GOT = 1.15

Virus hepatitis

GPT ↑

GPT/GOT ↓↓↓1

more than 2.5

chronic hepatitis

GPT ↑

GOT ↑

GPT/GOT = 1

Liver cancer, cirrhosis, Alcohol-induced hepatitis

GPT ↑

GOT ↑

GPT/GOT = 0.6~0.7

Accute myocardial infarct

GPT/GOT <1

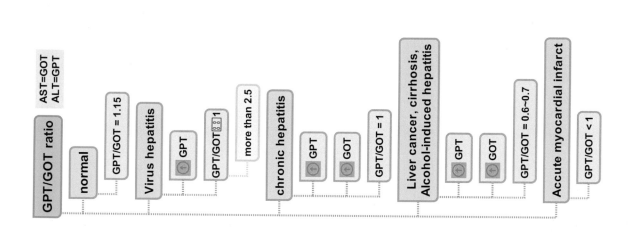

The AST/ALT ratio can provide important diagnostic clues

The normal AST/ALT ratio is approximately 0.8

The AST/ALT ratio of 2.0 or higher or ALT level exceeding 300 U/L may be indicative of alcoholic liver disease

The AST/ALT ratio is usually 1.0 or less in nonalcoholic fatty liver disease

Patients with a history of alcohol abuse but no significant alcoholic hepatitis or cirrhosis of the liver usually have an AST/ALT ratio less than 1.0

Patients with viral hepatitis, an AST/ALT ratio greater than 1.0 may be indicative of underlying cirrhosis with a high specificity (94–100%) but low sensitivity (44–75%)

Patients with Wilson's disease can show an AST/ALT ratio greater than 4.0

The liver

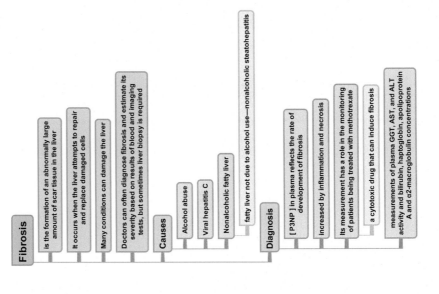

Fibrosis

- is the formation of an abnormally large amount of scar tissue in the liver
- It occurs when the liver attempts to repair and replace damaged cells
- Many conditions can damage the liver
- Doctors can often diagnose fibrosis and estimate its severity based on results of blood and imaging tests, but sometimes liver biopsy is required

Causes
- Alcohol abuse
- Viral hepatitis C
- Nonalcoholic fatty liver
  - fatty liver not due to alcohol use—nonalcoholic steatohepatitis

Diagnosis
- [P3NP] in plasma reflects the rate of development of fibrosis
- increased by inflammation and necrosis
- Its measurement has a role in the monitoring of patients being treated with methotrexate
- a cytotoxic drug that can induce fibrosis
- measurements of plasma GGT, AST, and ALT activity and bilirubin, haptoglobin, apolipoprotein A and α2-macroglobulin concentrations

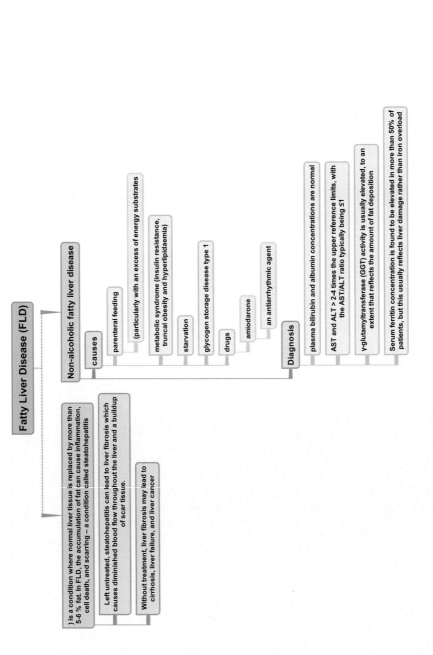

Fatty Liver Disease (FLD)

-) is a condition where normal liver tissue is replaced by more than 5-6 % fat. In FLD, the accumulation of fat can cause inflammation, cell death, and scarring – a condition called steatohepatitis
- Left untreated, steatohepatitis can lead to liver fibrosis which causes diminished blood flow throughout the liver and a buildup of scar tissue.
- Without treatment, liver fibrosis may lead to cirrhosis, liver failure, and liver cancer

Non-alcoholic fatty liver disease

causes
- parenteral feeding
  - (particularly with an excess of energy substrates
- metabolic syndrome (insulin resistance, truncal obesity and hyperlipidaemia)
- starvation
- glycogen storage disease type 1
- drugs
- amiodarone
  - an antiarrhythmic agent

Diagnosis
- plasma bilirubin and albumin concentrations are normal
- AST and ALT > 2-4 times the upper reference limits, with the AST/ALT ratio typically being ≤1
- γ-glutamyltransferase (GGT) activity is usually elevated, to an extent that reflects the amount of fat deposition
- Serum ferritin concentration is found to be elevated in more than 50% of patients, but this usually reflects liver damage rather than iron overload

42

The liver

The progression of liver disease

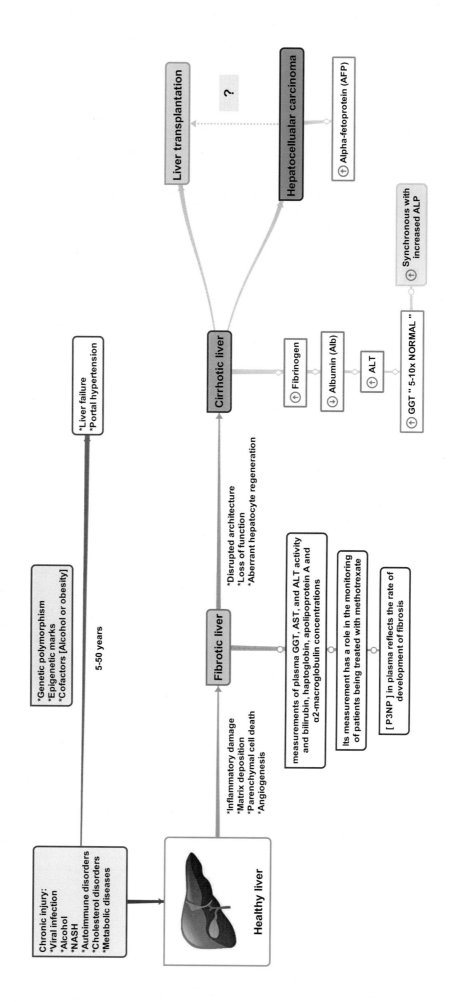

Chronic injury:
*Viral infection
*Alcohol
*NASH
*Autoimmune disorders
*Cholesterol disorders
*Metabolic diseases

*Genetic polymorphism
*Epigenetic marks
*Cofactors [Alcohol or obesity]

5-50 years

*Liver failure
*Portal hypertension

Healthy liver

*Inflammatory damage
*Matrix deposition
*Parenchymal cell death
*Angiogenesis

Fibrotic liver

*Disrupted architecture
*Loss of function
*Aberrant hepatocyte regeneration

Cirrhotic liver

Liver transplantation

?

Hepatocelluialar carcinoma

(↑) Alpha-fetoprotein (AFP)

measurements of plasma GGT, AST, and ALT activity and bilirubin, haptoglobin, apolipoprotein A and α2-macroglobulin concentrations

Its measurement has a role in the monitoring of patients being treated with methotrexate

[P3NP] in plasma reflects the rate of development of fibrosis

(↑) Fibrinogen

(↓) Albumin (Alb)

(↑) ALT

(↑) GGT " 5-10x NORMAL "

(↑) Synchronous with increased ALP

43

The kidneys

you will organize your knowledge about :

- The physiology of renal system
- The biochemical tests of renal functions
- The measurement of Glomerular Filtration Rate (GFR)
- The determination of creatinine clearance
- The classification of proteinuria
- The tubular function tests
- The Chronic renal failure (CRF)
- The Acute renal failure (ARF)

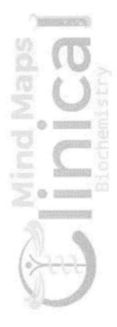

Mind Maps
Clinical
Biochemistry

44

The kidneys

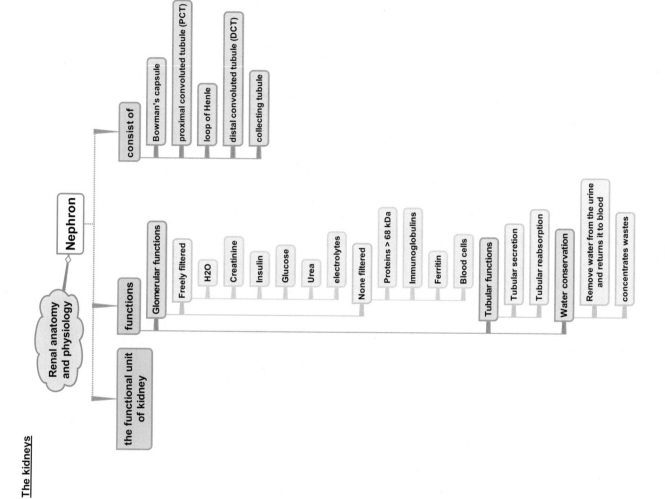

45

Nephron

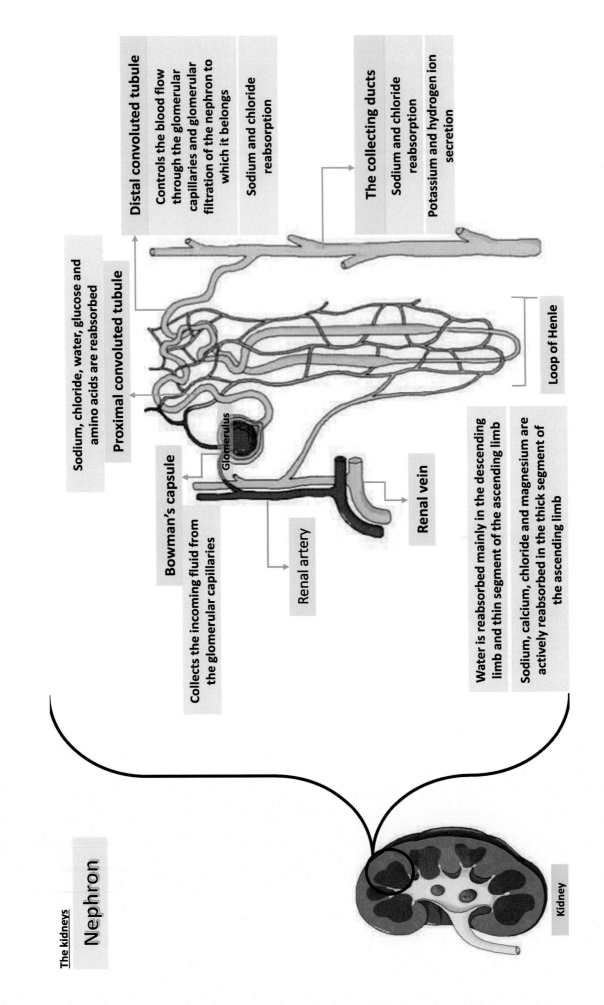

Distal convoluted tubule

Controls the blood flow through the glomerular capillaries and glomerular filtration of the nephron to which it belongs

Sodium and chloride reabsorption

The collecting ducts

Sodium and chloride reabsorption

Potassium and hydrogen ion secretion

Sodium, chloride, water, glucose and amino acids are reabsorbed

Proximal convoluted tubule

Glomerulus

Loop of Henle

Bowman's capsule

Collects the incoming fluid from the glomerular capillaries

Renal artery

Renal vein

Water is reabsorbed mainly in the descending limb and thin segment of the ascending limb

Sodium, calcium, chloride and magnesium are actively reabsorbed in the thick segment of the ascending limb

Kidney

46

The kidneys

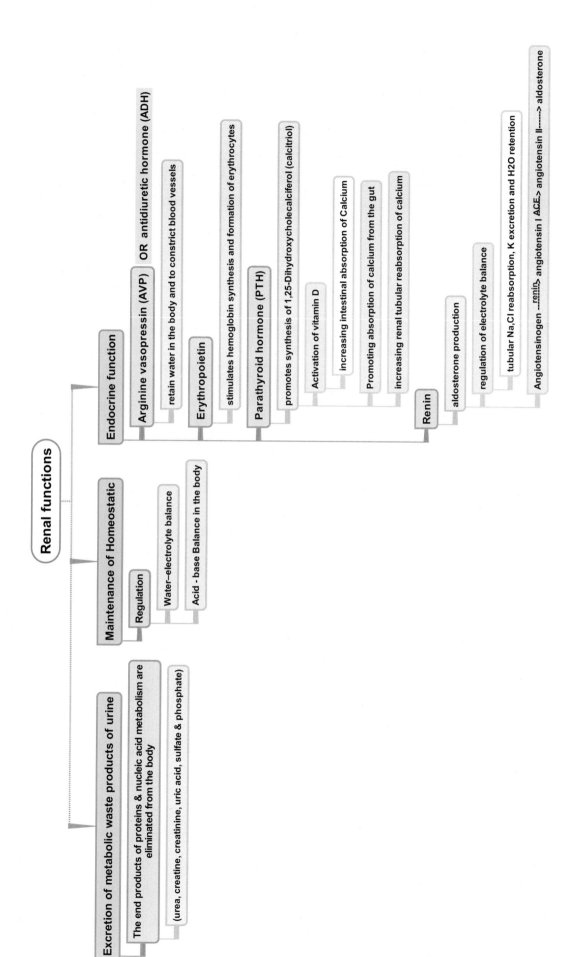

Renal functions

Excretion of metabolic waste products of urine

The end products of proteins & nucleic acid metabolism are eliminated from the body

(urea, creatine, creatinine, uric acid, sulfate & phosphate)

Maintenance of Homeostatic

Regulation

Water–electrolyte balance

Acid - base Balance in the body

Endocrine function

Arginine vasopressin (AVP)   OR antidiuretic hormone (ADH)

retain water in the body and to constrict blood vessels

Erythropoietin

stimulates hemoglobin synthesis and formation of erythrocytes

Parathyroid hormone (PTH)

promotes synthesis of 1,25-Dihydroxycholecalciferol (calcitriol)

Activation of vitamin D

increasing intestinal absorption of Calcium

Promoting absorption of calcium from the gut

increasing renal tubular reabsorption of calcium

Renin

aldosterone production

regulation of electrolyte balance

tubular Na,Cl reabsorption, K excretion and H2O retention

Angiotensinogen ....renin.... angiotensin I ..ACE..> angiotensin II ------> aldosterone

The kidneys

Endocrine links in the kidney

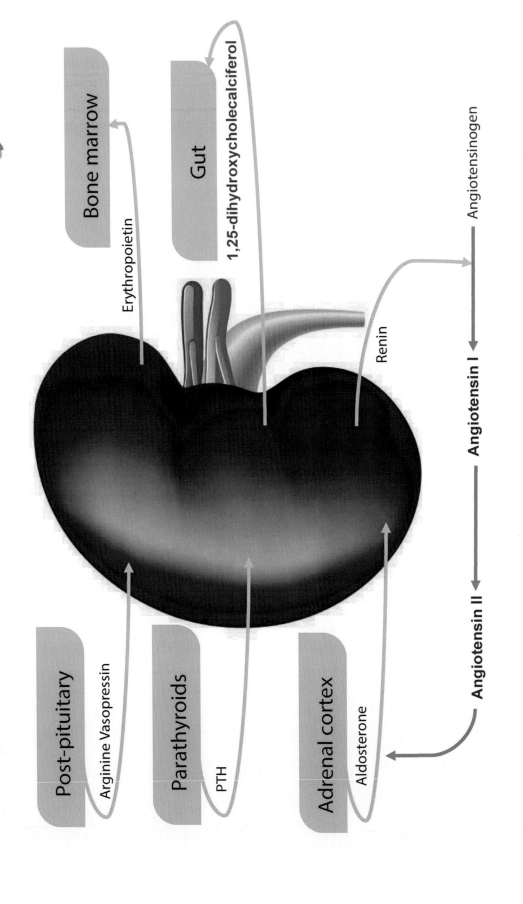

Bone marrow

Gut

1,25-dihydroxycholecalciferol

Erythropoietin

Post-pituitary

Arginine Vasopressin

Parathyroids

PTH

Adrenal cortex

Aldosterone

Renin

Angiotensinogen

Angiotensin I

Angiotensin II

48

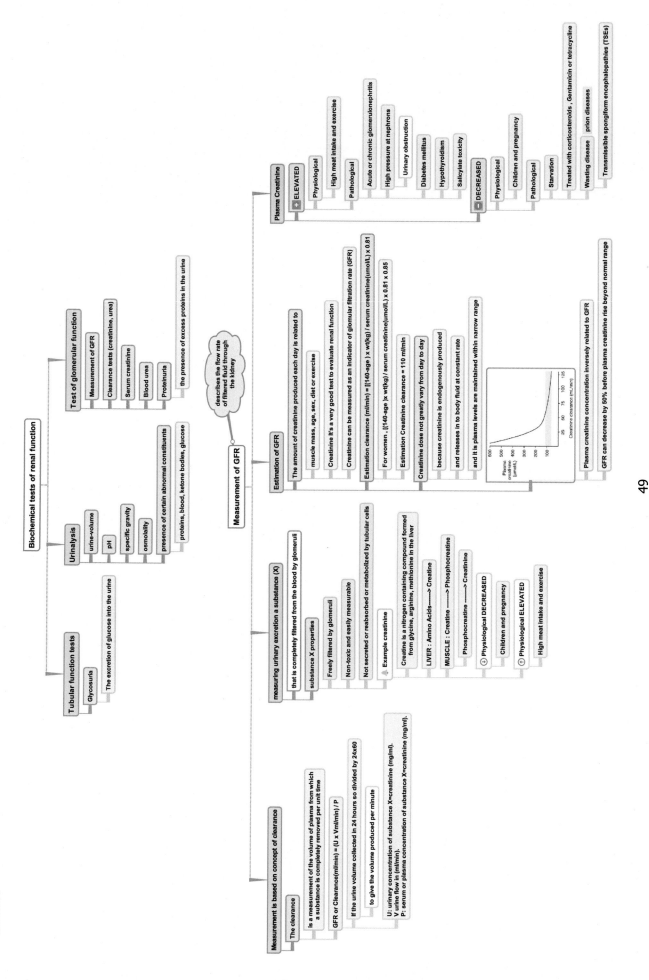

The kidneys

Biochemical tests of renal function

Tubular function tests
- Glycosuria
  - The excretion of glucose into the urine

Urinalysis
- urine-volume
- pH
- specific gravity
- osmolality
- presence of certain abnormal constituents
  - proteins, blood, ketone bodies, glucose

Test of glomerular function
- Measurement of GFR
- Clearance tests (creatinine, urea)
- Serum creatinine
- Blood urea
- Proteinuria
  - the presence of excess proteins in the urine

Measurement of GFR

(describes the flow rate of filtered fluid through the kidney)

Measurement is based on concept of clearance
- The clearance
  - is a measurement of the volume of plasma from which a substance is completely removed per unit time
- GFR or Clearance(ml/min) = (U x V ml/min) / P
- If the urine volume collected in 24 hours so divided by 24x60
  - to give the volume produced per minute
- U: urinary concentration of substance X=creatinine (mg/ml).
- V urine flow in (ml/min).
- P: serum or plasma concentration of substance X=creatinine (mg/ml).

measuring urinary excretion a substance (X)
- that is completely filtered from the blood by glomeruli
- substance X properties
  - Freely filtered by glomeruli
  - Non-toxic and easily measurable
  - Not secreted or reabsorbed or metabolized by tubular cells
- Example creatinine
  - Creatine is a nitrogen containing compound formed from glycine, arginine, methionine in the liver
  - LIVER : Amino Acids $\longrightarrow$ Creatine
  - MUSCLE : Creatine $\longrightarrow$ Phosphocreatine
  - Phosphocreatine $\longrightarrow$ Creatinine
  - (-) Physiological DECREASED
    - Children and pregnancy
  - (+) Physiological ELEVATED
    - High meat intake and exercise

Estimation of GFR
- The amount of creatinine produced each day is related to
  - muscle mass, age, sex, diet or exercise
- Creatinine it's a very good test to evaluate renal function
- Creatinine can be measured as an indicator of glomular filtration rate (GFR)
- Estimation clearance (ml/min) = [(140-age) x wt(kg) / serum creatinine(umol/L) x 0.81
- For women , [(140-age)x wt(kg) / serum creatinine(umol/L.) x 0.81 x 0.85
- Estimation Creatinine clearance = 110 ml/min
- Creatinine dose not greatly vary from day to day
  - because creatinine is endogenously produced
  - and releases in to body fluid at constant rate
  - and it is plasma levels are maintained within narrow range
- Plasma creatinine concentration inversely related to GFR
- GFR can decrease by 50% before plasma creatinine rise beyond normal range

Plasma Creatinine

ELEVATED (+)
- Physiological
  - High meat intake and exercise
- Pathological
  - Acute or chronic glomerulonephritis
  - High pressure at nephrons
  - Urinary obstruction
  - Diabetes mellitus
  - Hypothyroidism
  - Salicylate toxicity

DECREASED (-)
- Physiological
  - Children and pregnancy
- Pathological
  - Starvation
  - Treated with corticosteroids , Gentamicin or tetracycline
  - Wasting disease
  - prion diseases
  - Transmissible spongiform encephalopathies (TSEs)

49

The kidneys

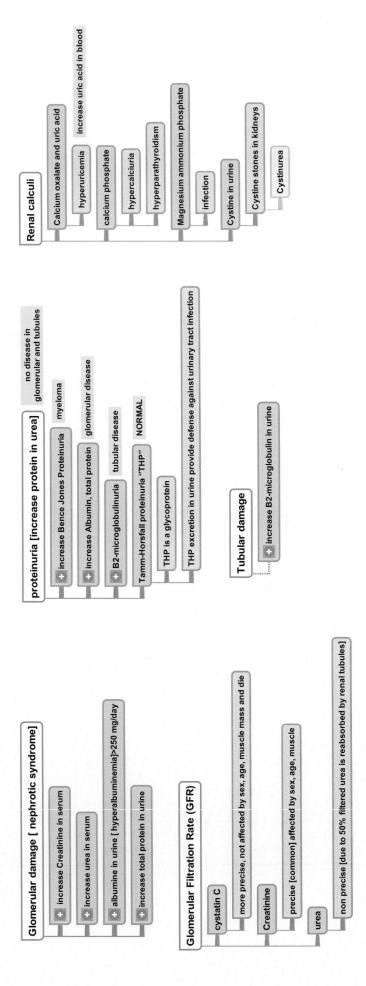

Glomerular damage [nephrotic syndrome]
- [+] increase Creatinine in serum
- [+] increase urea in serum
- albumine in urine [hyperalbuminemia]>250 mg/day
- [+] increase total protein in urine

Glomerular Filtration Rate (GFR)
- cystatin C — more precise, not affected by sex, age, muscle mass and die
- Creatinine — precise [common] affected by sex, age, muscle
- urea — non precise [due to 50% filtered urea is reabsorbed by renal tubules]

proteinuria [increase protein in urea]
- [+] increase Bence Jones Proteinuria — myeloma
- [+] increase Albumin, total protein — glomerular disease
- B2-microglobulinuria — tubular disease
- Tamm-Horsfall proteinuria ''THP'' — NORMAL
- THP is a glycoprotein
- THP excretion in urine provide defense against urinary tract infection
- no disease in glomerular and tubules

Tubular damage
- [+] increase B2-microglobulin in urine

Renal calculi
- Calcium oxalate and uric acid
- hyperuricemia — increase uric acid in blood
- calcium phosphate
- hypercalciuria
- hyperparathyroidism
- Magnesium ammonium phosphate
- infection
- Cystine in urine
- Cystine stones in kidneys
- Cystinurea

50

The kidneys

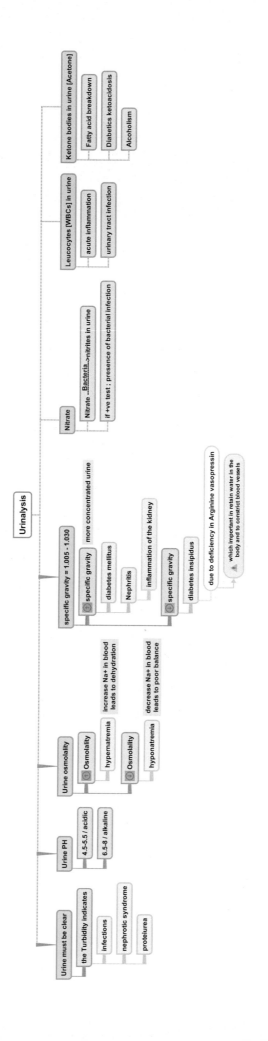

Urinalysis

Urine must be clear
- the Turbidity indicates
  - infections
  - nephrotic syndrome
  - proteiurea

Urine PH
- 4.5-5.5 / acidic
- 6.5-8 / alkaline

Urine osmolality
- ⊕ Osmolality
  - hypernatremia — increase Na+ in blood leads to dehydration
- ⊖ Osmolality
  - hyponatremia — decrease Na+ in blood leads to poor balance

specific gravity = 1.005 - 1.030
- ⊕ specific gravity — more concentrated urine
  - diabetes mellitus
  - Nephritis
  - inflammation of the kidney
- ⊖ specific gravity
  - diabetes insipidus
    - due to deficiency in Arginine vasopressin
    - ⚠ which important in retain water in the body and to constrict blood vessels

Nitrate
- Nitrate —Bacteria→nitrites in urine
- if +ve test ; presence of bacterial infection

Leucocytes [WBCs] in urine
- acute inflammation
- urinary tract infection

Ketone bodies in urine [Acetone]
- Fatty acid breakdown
- Diabetics ketoacidosis
- Alcoholism

51

The kidney

Renal Disorders

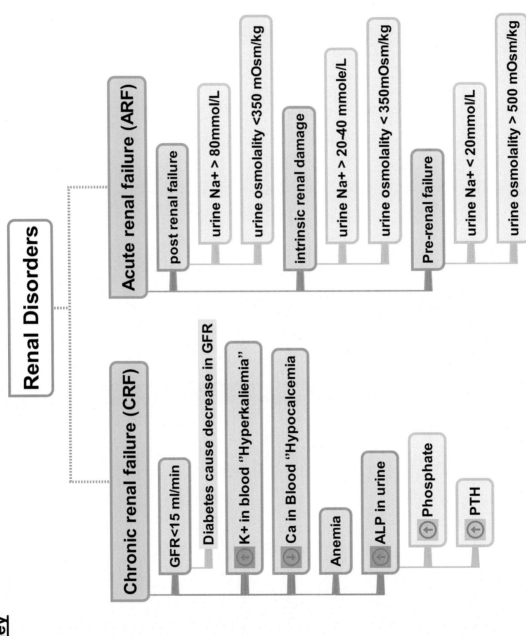

Chronic renal failure (CRF)
- GFR<15 ml/min
  - Diabetes cause decrease in GFR
- K+ in blood "Hyperkaliemia"
- Ca in Blood "Hypocalcemia"
- Anemia
- ALP in urine
  - Phosphate
  - PTH

Acute renal failure (ARF)
- post renal failure
  - urine Na+ > 80mmol/L
  - urine osmolality <350 mOsm/kg
- intrinsic renal damage
  - urine Na+ > 20-40 mmole/L
  - urine osmolality < 350mOsm/kg
- Pre-renal failure
  - urine Na+ <20mmol/L
  - urine osmolality > 500 mOsm/kg

Acute Kidney Injury

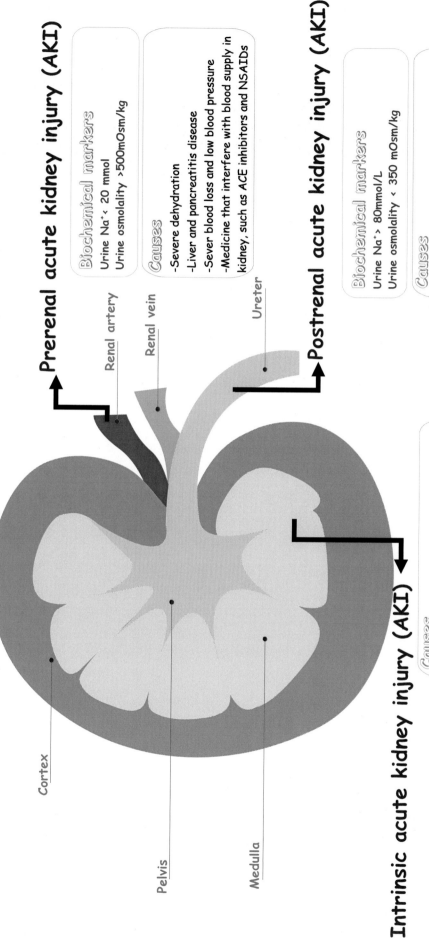

Prerenal acute kidney injury (AKI)

Biochemical markers
Urine Na+ < 20 mmol
Urine osmolality >500mOsm/kg

Causes
-Severe dehydration
-Liver and pancreatitis disease
-Sever blood loss and low blood pressure
-Medicine that interfere with blood supply in kidney, such as ACE inhibitors and NSAIDs

Postrenal acute kidney injury (AKI)

Biochemical markers
Urine Na+ > 80mmol/L
Urine osmolality < 350 mOsm/kg

Causes
-Kidney stones
-Benign prostatic hyperplasia BPH
-Neurogenic bladder
-Tubule obstruction
-Retroperitoneal fibrosis

Renal artery

Renal vein

Ureter

Cortex

Pelvis

Medulla

Intrinsic acute kidney injury (AKI)

Biochemical markers
Urine Na+ > 20-40 mmole/L
Urine osmolality < 350 mOsm/kg

Causes
-Acute glomerulonephritis (AGN)
-Interstitial nephritis
-Acute tubular necrosis
-Amyloidosis
-HUS/TTP (low blood platelet and red blood cell counts)

53

The **kidney**

How hypocalacemia and secondary hypoparathyrodisim develop in renal disease

Hypocalcaemia and hyperphosphatase

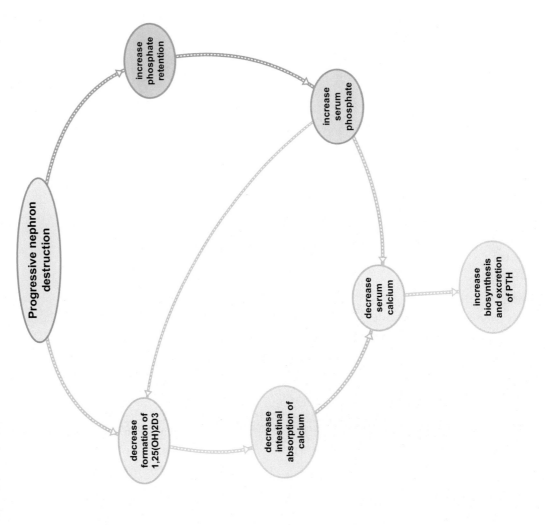

54

The kidney

an inherited disorder in which clusters of cysts develop primarily within kidneys

causing kidneys to enlarge and lose function over time

Cysts are noncancerous round sacs containing fluid

Having many cysts or large cysts can damage kidneys

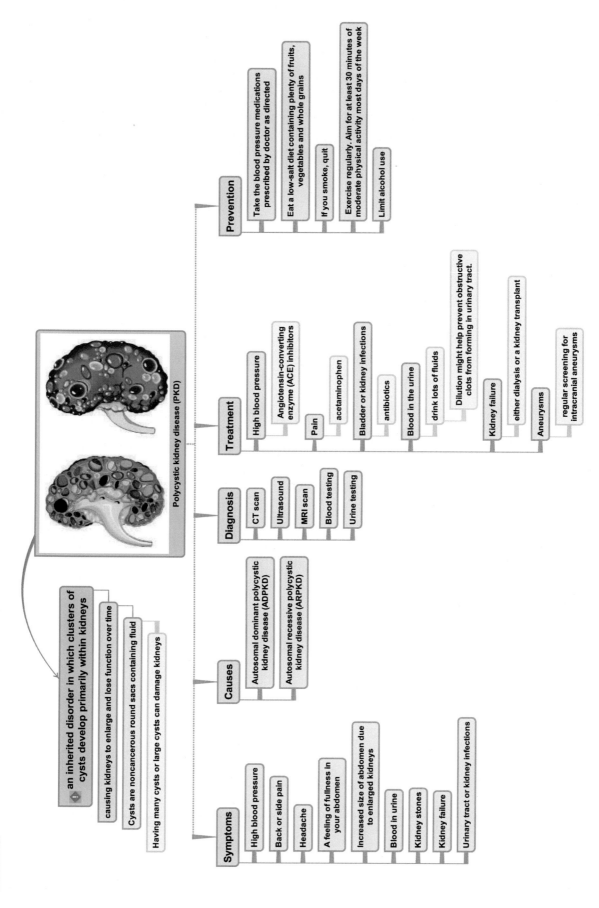

Polycystic kidney disease (PKD)

Symptoms
- High blood pressure
- Back or side pain
- Headache
- A feeling of fullness in your abdomen
- Increased size of abdomen due to enlarged kidneys
- Blood in urine
- Kidney stones
- Kidney failure
- Urinary tract or kidney infections

Causes
- Autosomal dominant polycystic kidney disease (ADPKD)
- Autosomal recessive polycystic kidney disease (ARPKD)

Diagnosis
- CT scan
- Ultrasound
- MRI scan
- Blood testing
- Urine testing

Treatment
- High blood pressure
- Angiotensin-converting enzyme (ACE) inhibitors
- Pain
- acetaminophen
- Bladder or kidney infections
- antibiotics
- Blood in the urine
- drink lots of fluids
- Dilution might help prevent obstructive clots from forming in urinary tract.
- Kidney failure
- either dialysis or a kidney transplant
- Aneurysms
- regular screening for intracranial aneurysms

Prevention
- Take the blood pressure medications prescribed by doctor as directed
- Eat a low-salt diet containing plenty of fruits, vegetables and whole grains
- If you smoke, quit
- Exercise regularly. Aim for at least 30 minutes of moderate physical activity most days of the week
- Limit alcohol use

55

The kidney

Kidney Stones

(renal lithiasis, nephrolithiasis) are hard deposits made of minerals and salts that form inside your kidneys

kidney stones

Symptoms
- Severe pain in the side and back, below the ribs
- Pain that radiates to the lower abdomen and groin
- Pain that comes in waves and fluctuates in intensity
- Pain on urination
- Pink, red or brown urine
- Cloudy or foul-smelling urine
- Nausea and vomiting
- Persistent need to urinate
- Urinating more often than usual
- Fever and chills if an infection is present
- Urinating small amounts

Types of kidney stones
- Calcium stones
  - Oxalate is a naturally occurring substance found in food and is also made daily by liver
  - Calcium stones may also occur in the form of calcium phosphate
  - more common in metabolic conditions, such as renal tubular acidosis
  - associated with certain migraine headaches or with taking certain seizure medications, such as topiramate (Topamax)
- Struvite stones
  - form in response to an infection, such as a urinary tract infection
  - These stones can grow quickly and become quite large
- Uric acid stones
  - form in people who don't drink enough fluids or who lose too much fluid
  - those who eat a high-protein diet, and those who have gout
- Cystine stones
  - in people with a hereditary disorder that causes the kidneys to excrete too much of certain amino acids (cystinuria)

Risk factors
- Family or personal history
- Dehydration
- ating a diet that's high in protein, sodium (salt) and sugar
- High body mass index (BMI), large waist size and weight gain
- Digestive diseases and surgery
  - Gastric bypass surgery, inflammatory bowel disease or chronic diarrhea
  - can cause changes in the digestive process that affect absorption of calcium and water
  - Increasing the levels of stone-forming substances in urine.
- renal tubular acidosis, cystinuria, hyperparathyroidism

Diagnosis
- Blood testing
- Urine testing
- X-rays
- Analysis of passed stones
  - to determine what's causing your kidney stones and to form a plan to prevent more kidney stones

Treatment
- Small stones with minimal symptoms
  - Drinking water
  - pain relievers such as ibuprofen
  - alpha blocker
    - relaxes the muscles in ureter, helping pass the kidney stone more quickly and with less pain
- Large stones and those that cause symptoms
  - Using sound waves to break up stones
    - extracorporeal shock wave lithotripsy (ESWL)
    - uses sound waves to create strong vibrations (shock waves) that break the stones into tiny pieces that can be passed in urine
  - Surgery to remove very large stones in the kidney
    - Using a scope to remove stones
  - Parathyroid gland surgery
    - Some calcium phosphate stones are caused by overactive parathyroid glands

Prevention
- Lifestyle changes
  - Drink water throughout the day
  - Eat fewer oxalate-rich foods
  - Choose a diet low in salt and animal protein
  - Continue eating calcium-rich foods, but use caution with calcium supplements

The kidneys

Urinary Tract Infections

Symptoms

- Pain or burning when one urinates
- An urge to urinate frequently and only passing small amounts of urine
- Inability to control urine release
- Pain or heavy feeling in lower abdomen
- Foul-smelling and/or cloudy urine
- Fever and chills
- Nausea and vomiting

Risk Factors

- Previous urinary tract infections
- Pregnancy
- Sexual activity, which can push bacteria into the urethra
- Use of feminine hygiene products that have deodorant
- Lack of estrogen, which allows bacteria that can cause urinary tract infections to grow more easily

Treatment

- Uncomplicated bladder infections
  - Antibiotics for 3-14 days depending on type
- In some cases
  - short hospitalization may be necessary
- Home treatment
  - A lot of water and fluids
  - Urinating frequently and emptying bladder fully

Prevention

- Make it a habit to drink plenty of fluids every day
- Do not hold in urine, but urinate as soon as you have the urge
- Empty bladder fully when urinating
- Cranberry juice or supplements and vitamin C may help in preventing future urinary tract infections

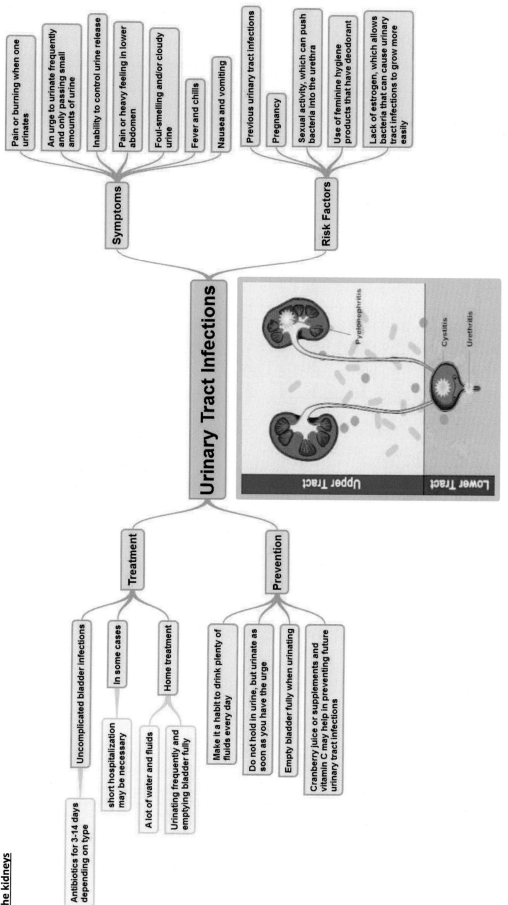

Upper Tract

Pyelonephritis

Cystitis

Urethritis

Lower Tract

57

The kidneys

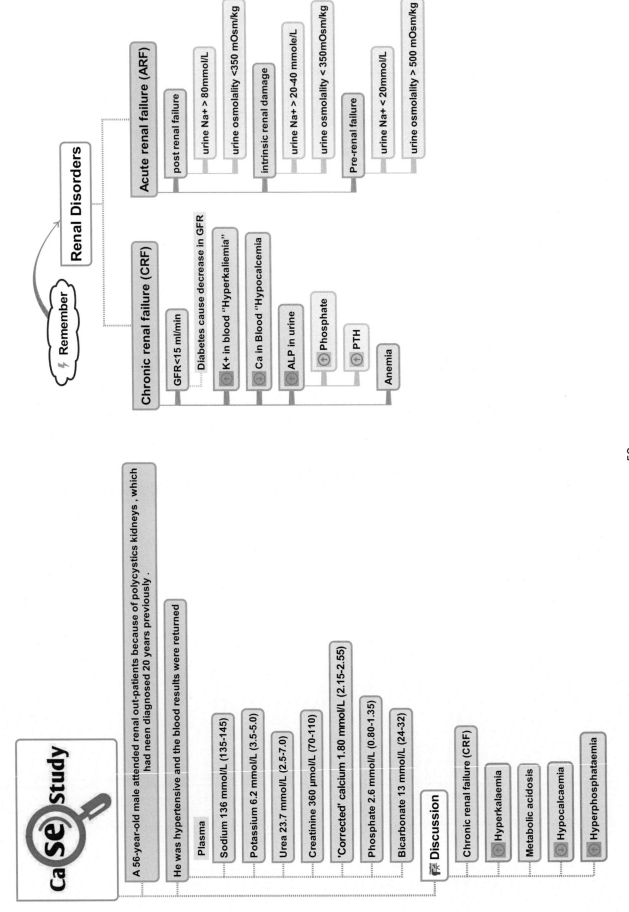

Renal Disorders

⚡ Remember

Acute renal failure (ARF)

- post renal failure
  - urine Na+ > 80mmol/L
  - urine osmolality <350 mOsm/kg
- intrinsic renal damage
  - urine Na+ > 20-40 mmole/L
  - urine osmolality < 350mOsm/kg
- Pre-renal failure
  - urine Na+ < 20mmol/L
  - urine osmolality > 500 mOsm/kg

Chronic renal failure (CRF)

- GFR<15 ml/min
  - Diabetes cause decrease in GFR
- K+ in blood "Hyperkaliemia"
- Ca in Blood "Hypocalcemia
- ALP in urine
- Phosphate
- PTH
- Anemia

Case Study

A 56-year-old male attended renal out-patients because of polycystics kidneys , which had neen diagnosed 20 years previously .

He was hypertensive and the blood results were returned

Plasma

- Sodium 136 mmol/L (135-145)
- Potassium 6.2 mmol/L (3.5-5.0)
- Urea 23.7 mmol/L (2.5-7.0)
- Creatinine 360 μmol/L (70-110)
- 'Corrected' calcium 1.80 mmol/L (2.15-2.55)
- Phosphate 2.6 mmol/L (0.80-1.35)
- Bicarbonate 13 mmol/L (24-32)

Discussion

- Chronic renal failure (CRF)
- Hyperkalaemia
- Metabolic acidosis
- Hypocalcaemia
- Hyperphosphataemia

58

The kidneys

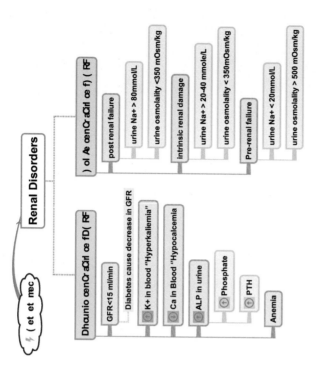

Renal Disorders

) ol Aᴇ cenⱰ aⱰᵗ œ f) (RF

- post renal failure
  - urine Na+ > 80mmol/L
  - urine osmolality <350 mOsm/kg
- Intrinsic renal damage
  - urine Na+ > 20-40 mmole/L
  - urine osmolality < 350mOsm/kg
- Pre-renal failure
  - urine Na+ < 20mmol/L
  - urine osmolality > 500 mOsm/kg

Dhᴄunio cenⱰ aⱰᵗ œ fD(RF

- GFR<15 ml/min
- Diabetes cause decrease in GFR
  - K+ in blood "Hyperkaliemia"
  - Ca in Blood "Hypocalcemia
  - ALP in urine
  - Phosphate
  - PTH
  - Anemia

⚡ (et et mec

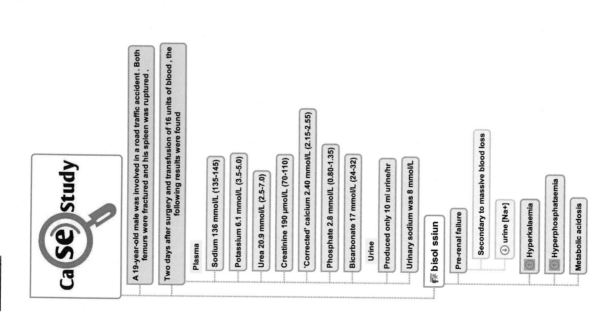

Case Study

A 19-year-old male was involved in a road traffic accident . Both femurs were fractured and his spleen was ruptured .

Two days after surgery and transfusion of 16 units of blood , the following results were found

Plasma
- Sodium 136 mmol/L (135-145)
- Potassium 6.1 mmol/L (3.5-5.0)
- Urea 20.9 mmol/L (2.5-7.0)
- Creatinine 190 µmol/L (70-110)
- 'Corrected' calcium 2.40 mmol/L (2.15-2.55)
- Phosphate 2.8 mmol/L (0.80-1.35)
- Bicarbonate 17 mmol/L (24-32)

Urine
- Produced only 10 ml urine/hr
- Urinary sodium was 8 mmol/L

bisol ssiun
- Pre-renal failure
  - Secondary to massive blood loss
    - urine [Na+]
    - Hyperkalaemia
    - Hyperphosphataemia
    - Metabolic acidosis

Disorder of carbohydrate metabolism

you will organize your knowledge about :

Glucose metabolism and diabetes mellitus

Diagnosis and monitory of diabetes mellitus

complication of Diabetes mellitus

Diabetic ketoacidosis

hypoglycemia

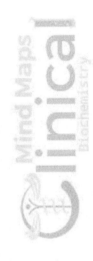
Clinical Mind Maps
Biochemistry

60

Disorder of carbohydrate metabolism

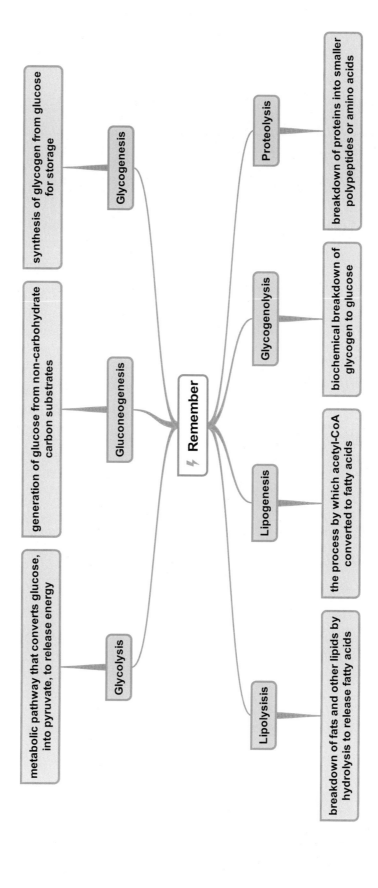

Disorder of carbohydrate metabolism

Insulin ⊖ **HYPOGLYCEMIA**

hormone produced by beta cells of the pancreatic islets

⊕ **increase**
- cellular glucose uptake
- glycogen synthesis
- protein synthesis
- fatty acid and TAG synthesis

⊖ **decrease**
- gluconeogenesis
- glycogenlysis
- lipolysis
- ketogenesis
- proteolysis

helps control blood glucose levels
- by signaling the liver and muscle and fat cells
- to take in glucose from the blood to be used for energy

Biosynthesis of insulin
- Insulin is a 51 amino acid polypeptide
- Secreted by β-cells of the pancreatic islets of Langerhans
- proinsulin cleavage to insulin and C-peptide

Cortisol

⊕ **Increase**
- gluconeogenesis
- glycogen synthesis
- proteolysis

⊖ **Decrease**
- tissue glucose utilization

⊕ **HYPERGLYCEMIA**

Growth Hormone

⊕ **increase**
- Glycogenlysis
- lipolysis

⊕ **HYPERGLYCEMIA**

Adrenaline

⊕ **increase**
- lipolysis
- glycogenlysis

⊕ **HYPERGLYCEMIA**

glucagon

⊕ **increase**
- glycogenlysis
- lipolysis
- gluconeogenesis
- ketogenesis

⊕ **HYPERGLYCEMIA**

62

Disorder of carbohydrate metabolism

Diabetes mellitus

is hyperglycaemia due to an insulin resistance and an absolute or relative lack of insulin

symptoms of diabetes

- Frequent urination
- Weakness
- Drowsiness
- Excessive thirst
- Blurred vision

prediabetes

(it is not high enough to be considered diabetes)

gestational diabetes

(temporary diabetes during pregnancy)

Hyperglycemia

high blood sugar is a condition in which an excessive amount of glucose circulates in the blood plasma

Plasma concentration 180mg/dL

Non-insulin-dependant diabetes mellitus (NIDDM)

(Diabetes mellitus type II)

- 85% of all diabetic patients
- 40-80 years of age
- Insulin resistance
  - cell are insulin-resistant and ignore its message to absorbed glucose
  - Reasons of resistance
    - Beta cell dysfunction
      - pancreas doesn't produce enough insulin
    - Environmental (stress)
    - Family history of diabetes
    - Obesity

Insulin-dependant diabetes mellitus (IDDM)

(Diabetes mellitus type I)

- 15% of all diabetic patients
- 9-15 years of age
- Abrupt onset
- insulin dependence
- Ketosis tendency
- lack of insulin due to
  - autoimmune destruction of insulin-production beta cells
  - environmental factors
    - as nitroso compounds
    - immune response to viral infection

Disorder of carbohydrate metabolism

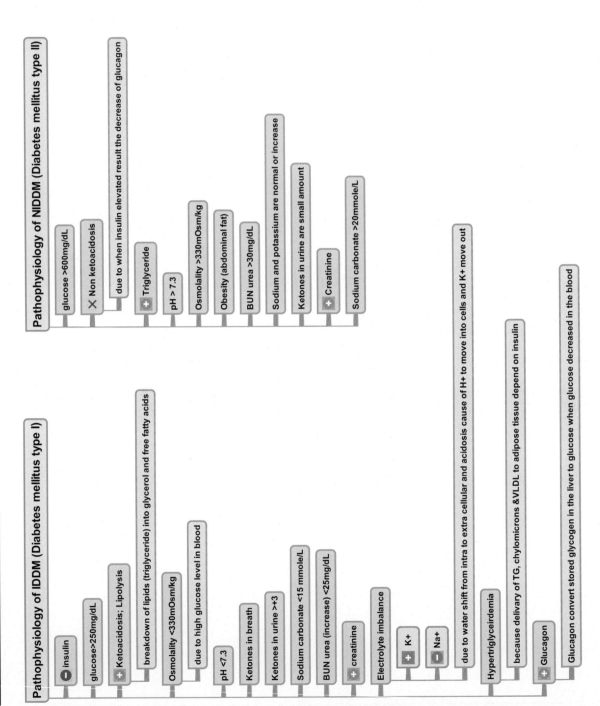

Pathophysiology of IDDM (Diabetes mellitus type I)

- ⊖ insulin
- glucose>250mg/dL
- ⊕ Ketoacidosis; Lipolysis
  - breakdown of lipids (triglyceride) into glycerol and free fatty acids
- Osmolality <330mOsm/kg
  - due to high glucose level in blood
- pH <7.3
- Ketones in breath
- Ketones in urine >+3
- Sodium carbonate <15 mmole/L
- BUN urea (increase) <25mg/dL
- ⊕ creatinine
- Electrolyte imbalance
- ⊕ K+
- ⊖ Na+
  - due to water shift from intra to extra cellular and acidosis cause of H+ to move into cells and K+ move out
- Hypertriglyceirdemia
  - because delivery of TG, chylomicrons &VLDL to adipose tissue depend on insulin
- ⊕ Glucagon
  - Glucagon convert stored glycogen in the liver to glucose when glucose decreased in the blood

Pathophysiology of NIDDM (Diabetes mellitus type II)

- glucose >600mg/dL
- ✗ Non ketoacidosis
  - due to when insulin elevated result the decrease of glucagon
- ⊕ Triglyceride
- pH > 7.3
- Osmolality >330mOsm/kg
- Obesity (abdominal fat)
- BUN urea >30mg/dL
- Sodium and potassium are normal or increase
- Ketones in urine are small amount
- ⊕ Creatinine
- Sodium carbonate >20mmole/L

Disorder of carbohydrate metabolism

Long term complication of Diabetes mellitus

Small blood vessels become weak, the blood flow is restricted and causes damage to tissues and organs

Microvascular complications

nephropathy
- leads ultimately to renal failure

neuropathy
- microangiopathy of nerve blood vessels and abnormal glucose metabolism in nerve cells

retinopathy
- lead to blindness because of vitreous haemorrhage from proliferating retinal vessels

Macrovascular disease
- related to atherosclerosis. Due to
- Increase formation of sorbitol by aldose reductase
- this cause osmotic damage and reduce the cellular myoinositol concentration
- Glucose react with amino groups in proteins to form Glycated plasma and tissue proteins
- leading to structural and functional damage
- Diabetes mellitus having high cholesterol, high triglyceride levels, and high blood pressure (hypertension)
- and all of these factors also contribute to heart disease

IDDM (Diabetes mellitus type I)
- [–] activity of lipoprotein lipase
- [+] VLDL, chylomicronaemia, triglyceride and LDL
- [–] HDL
- [+] risk cardiovascular disease

diabetes mellitus type II (NIDDM))
- [+] elevated glucose cause Glycation of apo B
- [–] reducing affinity of LDL receptor and increase atherosclerosis.
- [+] triglycerides and LDL
- [–] HDL
- [+] risk cardiovascular disease

<u>Disorder of carbohydrate metabolism</u>

EFFECTS OF DIABETES

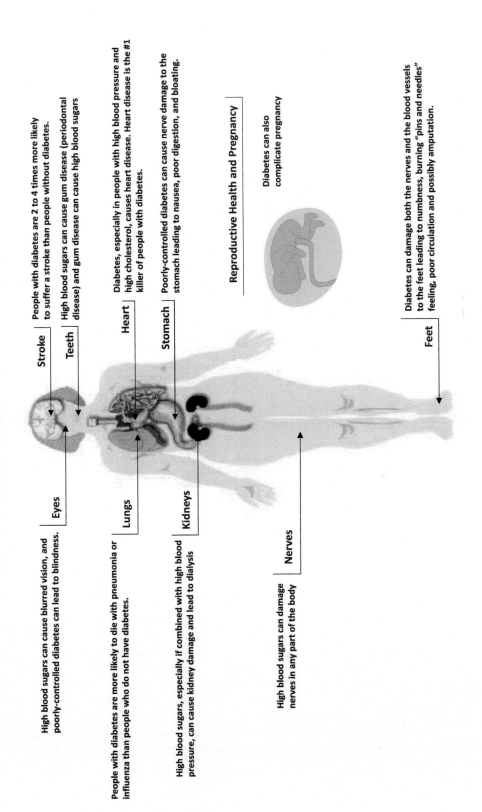

Stroke — People with diabetes are 2 to 4 times more likely to suffer a stroke than people without diabetes.

Teeth — High blood sugars can cause gum disease (periodontal disease) and gum disease can cause high blood sugars

Heart — Diabetes, especially in people with high blood pressure and high cholesterol, causes heart disease. Heart disease is the #1 killer of people with diabetes.

Stomach — Poorly-controlled diabetes can cause nerve damage to the stomach leading to nausea, poor digestion, and bloating.

Reproductive Health and Pregnancy

Diabetes can also complicate pregnancy

Feet — Diabetes can damage both the nerves and the blood vessels to the feet leading to numbness, burning "pins and needles" feeling, poor circulation and possibly amputation.

Eyes — High blood sugars can cause blurred vision, and poorly-controlled diabetes can lead to blindness.

Lungs — People with diabetes are more likely to die with pneumonia or influenza than people who do not have diabetes.

Kidneys — High blood sugars, especially if combined with high blood pressure, can cause kidney damage and lead to dialysis

Nerves — High blood sugars can damage nerves in any part of the body

66

Disorder of carbohydrate metabolism

TYPES OF DIABETIC NEUROPATHY

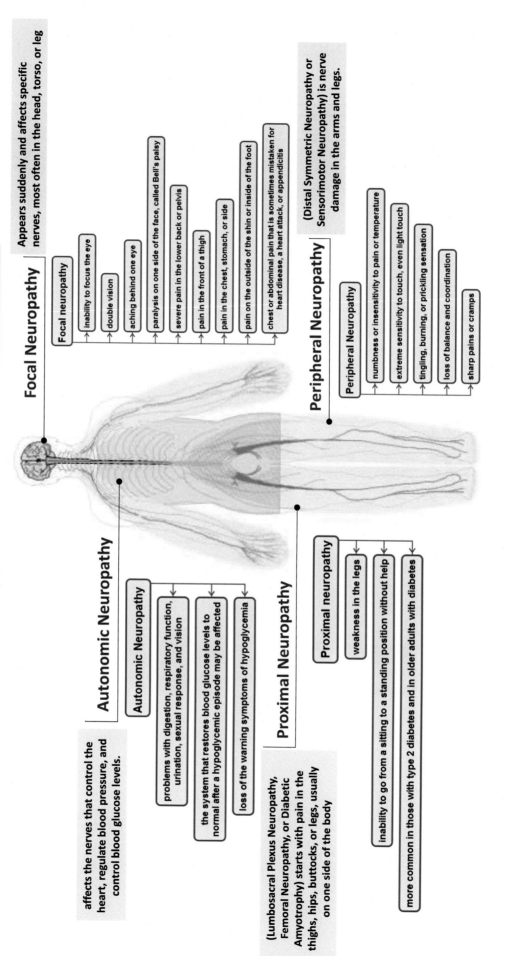

Focal Neuropathy

Appears suddenly and affects specific nerves, most often in the head, torso, or leg

Focal neuropathy

- inability to focus the eye
- double vision
- aching behind one eye
- paralysis on one side of the face, called Bell's palsy
- severe pain in the lower back or pelvis
- pain in the front of a thigh
- pain in the chest, stomach, or side
- pain on the outside of the shin or inside of the foot
- chest or abdominal pain that is sometimes mistaken for heart disease, a heart attack, or appendicitis

Peripheral Neuropathy

(Distal Symmetric Neuropathy or Sensorimotor Neuropathy) is nerve damage in the arms and legs.

Peripheral Neuropathy

- numbness or insensitivity to pain or temperature
- extreme sensitivity to touch, even light touch
- tingling, burning, or prickling sensation
- loss of balance and coordination
- sharp pains or cramps

Autonomic Neuropathy

affects the nerves that control the heart, regulate blood pressure, and control blood glucose levels.

Autonomic Neuropathy

- problems with digestion, respiratory function, urination, sexual response, and vision
- the system that restores blood glucose levels to normal after a hypoglycemic episode may be affected
- loss of the warning symptoms of hypoglycemia

Proximal Neuropathy

(Lumbosacral Plexus Neuropathy, Femoral Neuropathy, or Diabetic Amyotrophy) starts with pain in the thighs, hips, buttocks, or legs, usually on one side of the body

Proximal neuropathy

- weakness in the legs
- inability to go from a sitting to a standing position without help
- more common in those with type 2 diabetes and in older adults with diabetes

67

Disorder of carbohydrate metabolism

DIABETES RISK FACTORS

Inactivity

Pregnancy

High
Cholesterol

Obesity

Family
History

Certain
Medications

Race

Hypertension

Stress

Age

Disorder of carbohydrate metabolism

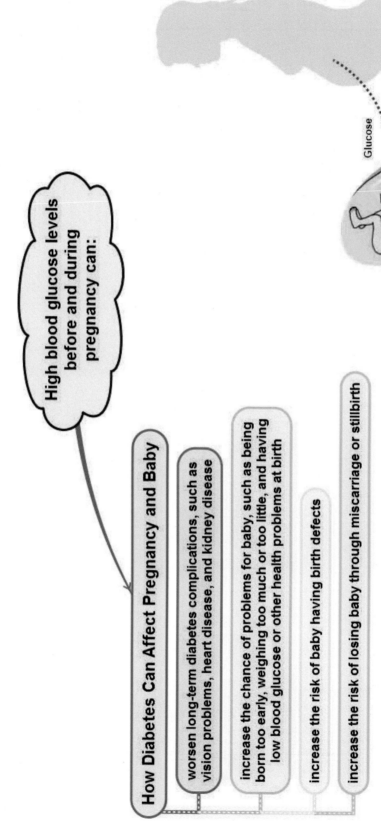

High blood glucose levels before and during pregnancy can:

How Diabetes Can Affect Pregnancy and Baby

worsen long-term diabetes complications, such as vision problems, heart disease, and kidney disease

increase the chance of problems for baby, such as being born too early, weighing too much or too little, and having low blood glucose or other health problems at birth

increase the risk of baby having birth defects

increase the risk of losing baby through miscarriage or stillbirth

Glucose

Disorder of carbohydrate metabolism

Diabetic Retinopathy

is the most common diabetic eye disease and a leading cause of blindness in American adults. It is caused by changes in the blood vessels of the retina

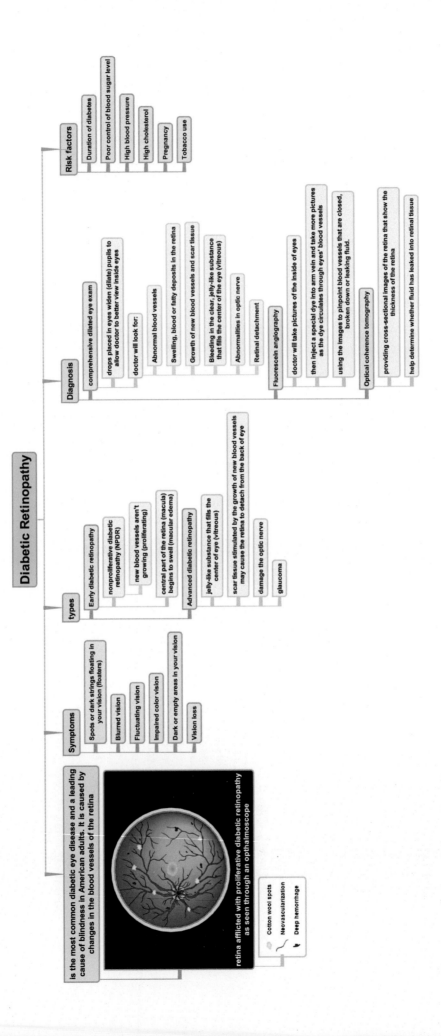

retina afflicted with proliferative diabetic retinopathy as seen through an opthalmoscope

Cotton wool spots
Neovascularization
Deep hemorrhage

Symptoms
- Spots or dark strings floating in your vision (floaters)
- Blurred vision
- Fluctuating vision
- Impaired color vision
- Dark or empty areas in your vision
- Vision loss

types
- Early diabetic retinopathy
- nonproliferative diabetic retinopathy (NPDR)
  - new blood vessels aren't growing (proliferating)
  - central part of the retina (macula) begins to swell (macular edema)
- Advanced diabetic retinopathy
  - jelly-like substance that fills the center of eye (vitreous)
  - scar tissue stimulated by the growth of new blood vessels may cause the retina to detach from the back of eye
  - damage the optic nerve
  - glaucoma

Diagnosis
- comprehensive dilated eye exam
  - drops placed in eyes widen (dilate) pupils to allow doctor to better view inside eyes
  - doctor will look for:
    - Abnormal blood vessels
    - Swelling, blood or fatty deposits in the retina
    - Growth of new blood vessels and scar tissue
    - Bleeding in the clear, jelly-like substance that fills the center of the eye (vitreous)
    - Abnormalities in optic nerve
    - Retinal detachment
- Fluorescein angiography
  - doctor will take pictures of the inside of eyes
  - then inject a special dye into arm vein and take more pictures as the dye circulates through eyes' blood vessels
  - using the images to pinpoint blood vessels that are closed, broken down or leaking fluid.
- Optical coherence tomography
  - providing cross-sectional images of the retina that show the thickness of the retina
  - help determine whether fluid has leaked into retinal tissue

Risk factors
- Duration of diabetes
- Poor control of blood sugar level
- High blood pressure
- High cholesterol
- Pregnancy
- Tobacco use

Disorder of carbohydrate metabolism

Diabetes and Foot Problems

High blood glucose from diabetes causes two problems that can hurt feet:

Nerve damage:

With damaged nerves, you might not feel pain, heat, or cold in your legs and feet

A sore or cut on your foot may get worse because you do not know it is there

This lack of feeling is caused by nerve damage, also called diabetic neuropathy

Nerve damage can lead to a sore or an infection.

Poor blood flow

peripheral vascular disease, also called PVD

Poor blood flow makes it hard for a sore or infection to hea

moking when you have diabetes makes blood flow problems much worse.

Diabetes and Dental Disease

High blood glucose can make tooth and gum problems worse

Smoking makes it more likely to get a bad case of gum disease, especially if have diabetes and are age 45 or older

Red, sore, and bleeding gums are the first sign of gum disease

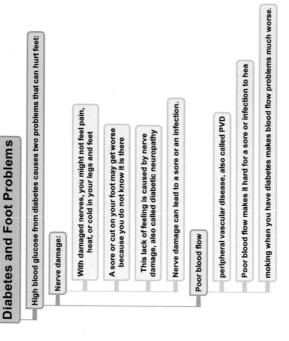

lead to periodontitis

Periodontitis is an infection in the gums and the bone that holds the teeth in place

If the infection gets worse, gums may pull away from teeth, making teeth look long

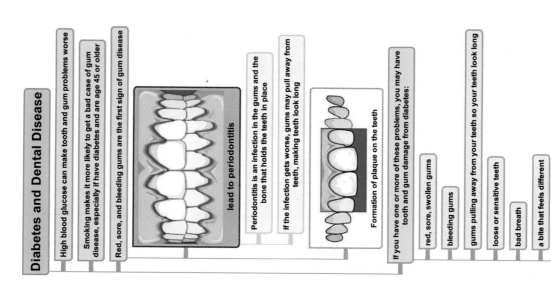

Formation of plaque on the teeth

If you have one or more of these problems, you may have tooth and gum damage from diabetes:

red, sore, swollen gums

bleeding gums

gums pulling away from your teeth so your teeth look long

loose or sensitive teeth

bad breath

a bite that feels different

dentures—false teeth—that do not fit well

Disorder of carbohydrate metabolism

Hypoglycemia

blood glucose decreases to below normal levels.

(glucose below 2.2mmole/L OR glucose below 40mg/dL)

Reactive hypoglycaemia (postprandial hypoglycemia)

- insulin-induced
  - Inappropriate or excessive insulin predictably
- Drug-induced
  - salicylate, paracetamol and β-blockers (effect of adrenaline)
- Alcohol
  - Mechanisms include inhibition of gluconeogenesis, malnutrition and liver disease

Fasting hypoglycaemia (postabsorptive hypoglycemia)

- Insulinoma
  - is a tumor of the pancreas that produces excessive amounts of insulin
- Malignancy.
- Hepatic and renal disease
- Addison's disease
  - (hypoglycaemia is occasionally a feature of adrenal insufficiency
- Sepsis
  - cytokines stimulate insulin secretion

72

Disorder of carbohydrate metabolism

diagnosis of diabetes mellitus

Fasting plasma glucose

- (10-16 hr) ≥126mg/dl (7mmole/L)

Urinary ketones

- ketone bodies are present in the urine because using an alternative source of energy
- (acetoacetate, beta-hydroxybutyrate)
  - type I diabetes mellitus

Glycated haemoglobin (Hemoglobin A1c (HbA1c) in human blood)

- for evaluation of glycemic control in diabetes mellitus
- HbA1c provide an indication of glucose levels over the preceding 4-8 weeks
- formed continuously by the adduction of glucose to the N-terminal of the hemoglobin beta chain
- HbA1c in diabetic subjects to be elevated 2-3 fold over the levels found in normal individuals
- as an indicator of metabolic control of the diabetic
- The non-glycosylated hemoglobin, which consists of the bulk of the hemoglobin has been designated HbA0
- The present procedure utilizes a antigen and antibody reaction to directly determine the concentration of the HbA1c

Oral glucose tolerance test

- Use to diagnostic of NIDDM and gestational diabetes
- 1.Patient should eat normal diet, containing at least 250 g CHO/ day , for 3 days
- 2.then the sample taken after fasting over night
- 3.then the patient is given 75 g of glucose
- 4.after that blood is taken each 30 minutes for 2 hours
  - glucose ≥200mg/dl (11.1mmole/L)
    - diabetes mellitus
  - glucose 140-200(7.8-11.1mmole/L)
    - glucose intolerance

Insulin C-peptide test

- indicates how much insulin is being produced
- used to monitor insulin production in the body
- Its ability to determine the cause of low blood sugar or distinguish between type 1 and type 2 diabetes
- insulin C-peptide admiration to distinguish endogenous insulin from exogenou
- C-peptide is more reliable marker for endogenous insulin secretion

73

Disorder of carbohydrate metabolism

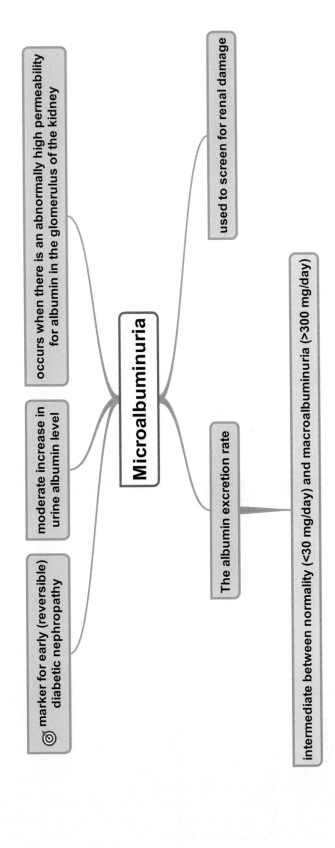

- marker for early (reversible) diabetic nephropathy
- moderate increase in urine albumin level
- occurs when there is an abnormally high permeability for albumin in the glomerulus of the kidney
- used to screen for renal damage

Microalbuminuria

The albumin excretion rate

intermediate between normality (<30 mg/day) and macroalbuminuria (>300 mg/day)

74

Disorder of carbohydrate metabolism

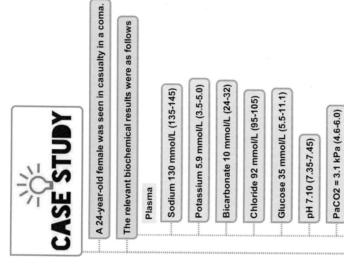

CASE STUDY

A 24-year-old female was seen in casualty in a coma.

The relevant biochemical results were as follows

Plasma

Sodium 130 mmol/L (135-145)

Potassium 5.9 mmol/L (3.5-5.0)

Bicarbonate 10 mmol/L (24-32)

Chloride 92 mmol/L (95-105)

Glucose 35 mmol/L (5.5-11.1)

pH 7.10 (7.35-7.45)

PaCO2 = 3.1 kPa (4.6-6.0)

PaO2 = 11.1 kPa (9.3-13.3)

Discussion

type 1 diabetes mellitus

diabetic ketoacidosis

hyperglycaemia

hyponatraemia

hyperkalaemia

metabolic acidosis

75

Lipids, lipoproteins and cardiovascular disease

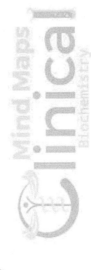

Mind Maps
Clinical
Biochemistry

you will organize your knowledge about :

The types and functions of lipids

The types and functions of Apolipoprotein

The metabolism pathway of HDL , LDL , VLDL and Chylomicrons

The causes of primary and secondary hyperlipidemia

Lipids, lipoproteins and cardiovascular disease

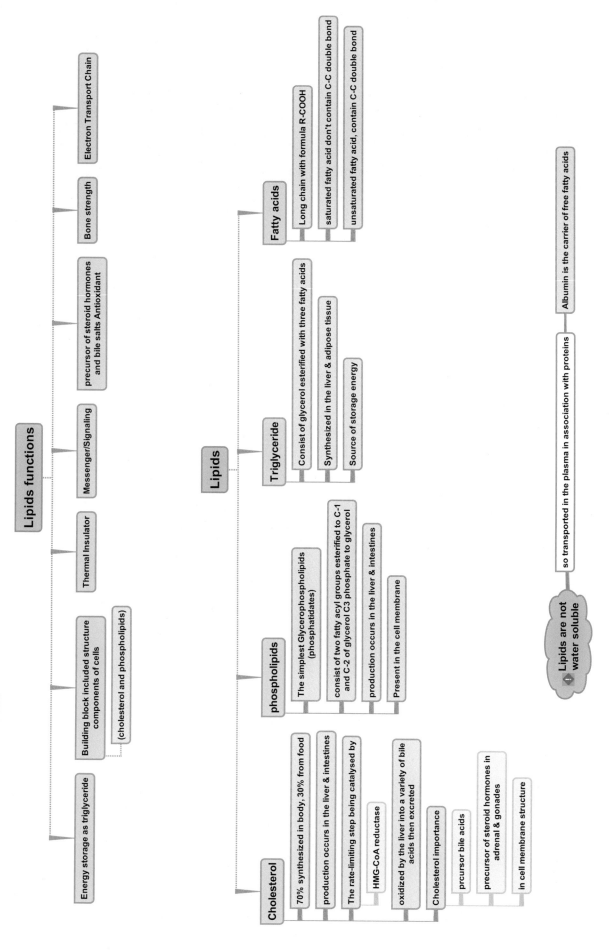

Lipids functions

- Energy storage as triglyceride
- Building block included structure components of cells
  - (cholesterol and phospholipids)
- Thermal Insulator
- Messenger/Signaling
- precursor of steroid hormones and bile salts Antioxidant
- Bone strength
- Electron Transport Chain

Lipids

Fatty acids
- Long chain with formula R-COOH
- saturated fatty acid don't contain C-C double bond
- unsaturated fatty acid, contain C-C double bond

Triglyceride
- Consist of glycerol esterified with three fatty acids
- Synthesized in the liver & adipose tissue
- Source of storage energy

phospholipids
- The simplest Glycerophospholipids (phosphatidates)
- consist of two fatty acyl groups esterified to C-1 and C-2 of glycerol C3 phosphate to glycerol
- production occurs in the liver & intestines
- Present in the cell membrane

Cholesterol
- 70% synthesized in body, 30% from food
- production occurs in the liver & intestines
- The rate-limiting step being catalysed by
  - HMG-CoA reductase
- oxidized by the liver into a variety of bile acids then excreted
- Cholesterol importance
  - prcursor bile acids
  - precursor of steroid hormones in adrenal & gonades
  - in cell membrane structure

Lipids are not water soluble
- so transported in the plasma in association with proteins
  - Albumin is the carrier of free fatty acids

77

Lipids, lipoproteins and cardiovascular disease

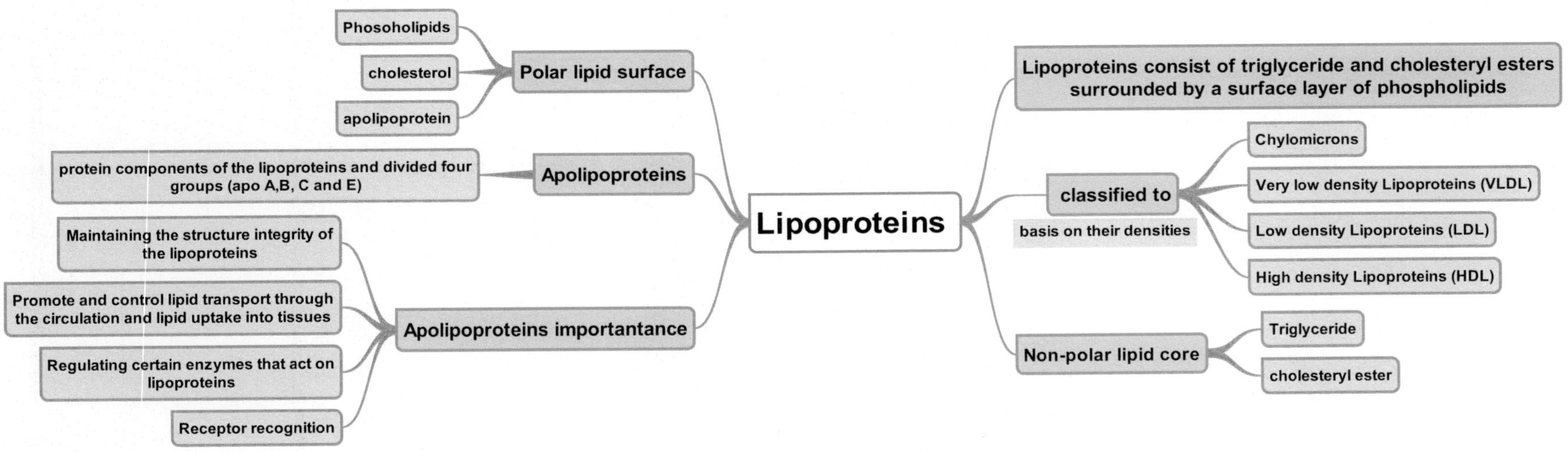

Lipoproteins

Lipoproteins consist of triglyceride and cholesteryl esters surrounded by a surface layer of phospholipids

classified to
basis on their densities
- Chylomicrons
- Very low density Lipoproteins (VLDL)
- Low density Lipoproteins (LDL)
- High density Lipoproteins (HDL)

Non-polar lipid core
- Triglyceride
- cholesteryl ester

Polar lipid surface
- Phosoholipids
- cholesterol
- apolipoprotein

Apolipoproteins
- protein components of the lipoproteins and divided four groups (apo A,B, C and E)

Apolipoproteins importantance
- Maintaining the structure integrity of the lipoproteins
- Promote and control lipid transport through the circulation and lipid uptake into tissues
- Regulating certain enzymes that act on lipoproteins
- Receptor recognition

78

Lipids, lipoproteins and cardiovascular disease

Apolipoproteins

Apolipoprotein A (apo A)

Apo A-I
- the major protein component of high-density lipoprotein HDL
- Deficiency of apo A1 is associated with HDL deficiencies
- Tangier disease and systemic non-neuropathic amyloidosis
- activate LCAT structural in HDL

Apo A-II
- Is a protein that in humans is encoded by the APOA2 gene
- Inhibit HTGL at high concentration structural in HDL

Apolipoprotein B (apo B)

apo B-100
- structural in LDL and VLDL receptor binding
- Mutations (changes) in apo B-100 can cause familial hypercholesterolemia
- form of high cholesterol that is passed down in families (inherited)

Apolipoprotein C (apo C)

Apo C-2
- activates lipoprotein lipase
- Defective apo C2 production
- causes hyperlipoproteinaemia type IB
- hypertriglyceridaemia, xanthomas and increased risk of pancreatitis and early atherosclerosis

Apo C-3
- inhibits lipoprotein lipase and hepatic lipase
- inhibits clearance of CM and VLDL remnant particle
- ◆ Serum levels of apo C1 and apo C3 are reduced in patients with stomach cancer

Apolipoprotein E (apo E)
- binding to LDL and remnant receptor
- involved in receptor recognition of intermediate-density lipoprotein and chylomicron remnant by the liver
- In familial dysbetalipoproteinaemia
- increased plasma cholesterol and triglycerides are the consequence of impaired clearance of chylomicron and VLDL remnants because of a defect in apo E

Apolipoprotein D (apo D)
- component of HDL in human plasma
- biomarker of androgen insensitivity syndrome
- is increasing evidence for a prominent neuroprotective role of apo D because of its antioxidant and anti-inflammatory activity

Apolipoprotein H (apo H)
- called glycoprotein I, beta-2 (B2gp1)
- has been implicated in a variety of physiological processes
- blood coagulation
- haemostasis
- production of antiphospholipid antibodies characteristic of antiphospholipid syndrome

Apolipoproteins

79

Lipids, lipoproteins and cardiovascular disease

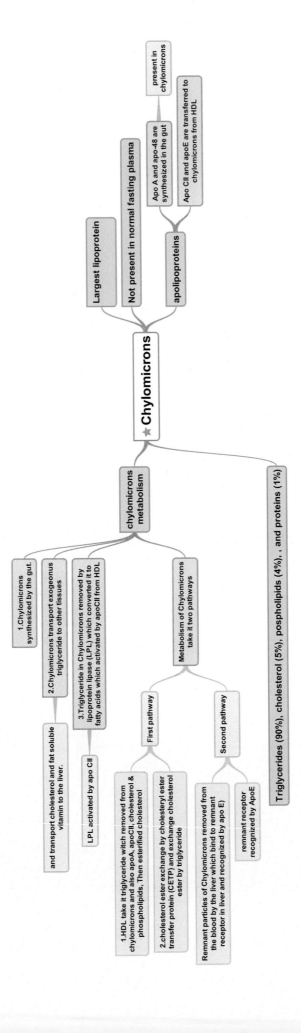

Chylomicrons

Largest lipoprotein

Not present in normal fasting plasma

apolipoproteins

Apo A and apo-48 are synthesized in the gut

present in chylomicrons

Apo CII and apoE are transferred to chylomicrons from HDL

chylomicrons metabolism

1.Chylomicrons synthesized by the gut.

2.Chylomicrons transport exogeonus triglyceride to other tissues

and transport cholesterol and fat soluble vitamin to the liver.

3.Triglyceride in Chylomicrons removed by lipoprotein lipase (LPL) which converted it to fatty acids which activated by apoCII from HDL

LPL activated by apo CII

Metabolism of Chylomicrons take it two pathways

First pathway

1.HDL take it triglyceride witch removed from chylomicrons and also apoA, apoCII, cholesterol & phospholipids, Then esterified cholesterol

2.cholesterol ester exchange by cholesteryl ester transfer protein (CETP) and exchange cholesterol ester by triglyceride

Second pathway

Remnant particles of Chylomicrons removed from the blood by the liver which bind to remnant receptor in liver and recognized by apo E)

remnant receptor recognized by ApoE

Triglycerides (90%), cholesterol (5%), pospholipids (4%), , and proteins (1%)

80

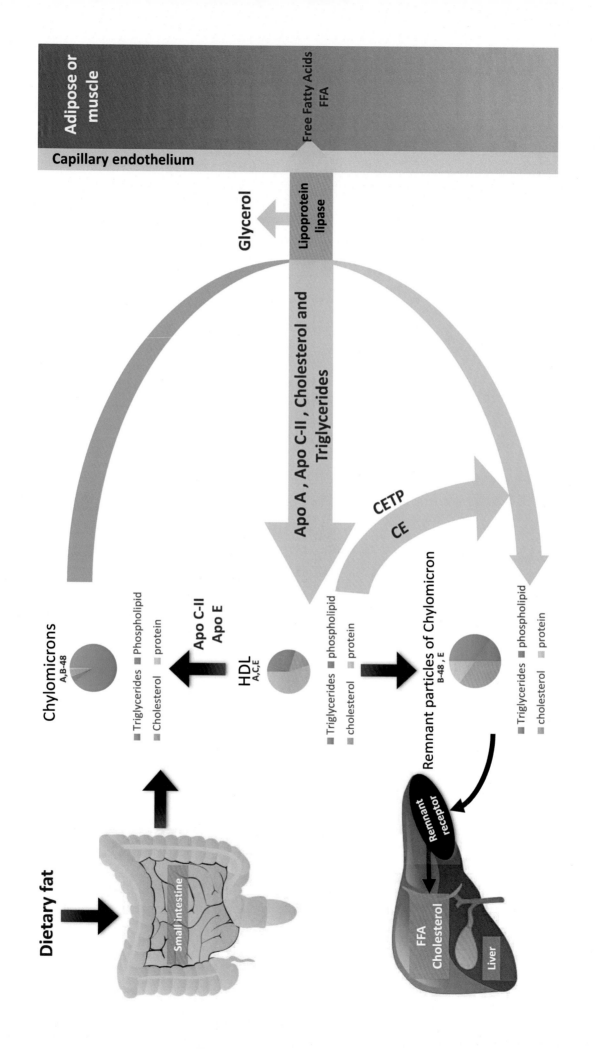

★ **Very Low Density Lipoproteins (VLDL) Metabolism**

- VLDL in synthesized in liver and transport endogenous triglyceride from liver to other tissue
- VLDL in triglyceride removed by lipoprotein lipase (LPL)
- At the same time, cholesterol, phospholipids, apo C, apo E transferred to HDL.
- SO VLDL convert to IDL
- Cholesterol esterified by (CETP) in HDL and exchange it with triglyceride in IDL
- Some IDL removed by liver by LDL receptor in the liver
- Most IDL removed by hepatic triglyceride lipase and converted to LDL

★ **Low density Lipoproteins (LDL) or bad cholesterol**

⊕ Main carrier of cholesterol from liver to peripheral tissues

⊕ LDL in blood associated with atherosclerosis, heart disease and myocardial infraction.why
- 1.LDL cholesterol is easy to stick to the walls of blood vessels
- 2.high LDL in blood will deposited in blood artery and trigger clot formation

Metabolism of LDL
- 1. LDL uptake by liver and other tissue by recognition of apoB-100 in LDL by the LDL receptor
- 2. LDL hydrolysed by lysosomal enzymes releasing free cholesterol

So Free cholesterol results
- ➊ Inhibit HMG-COA reductase which cause decease cholesterol synthesis
- ➋ Inhibit LDL receptor synthesis
- ⊕ Stimulates cholesterol esterification by the enzyme acyl CoA: cholesterol acyl transferase (ACAT)

⊕ Rich in cholesterol

⊕ Generated from VLDL in the circulation

82

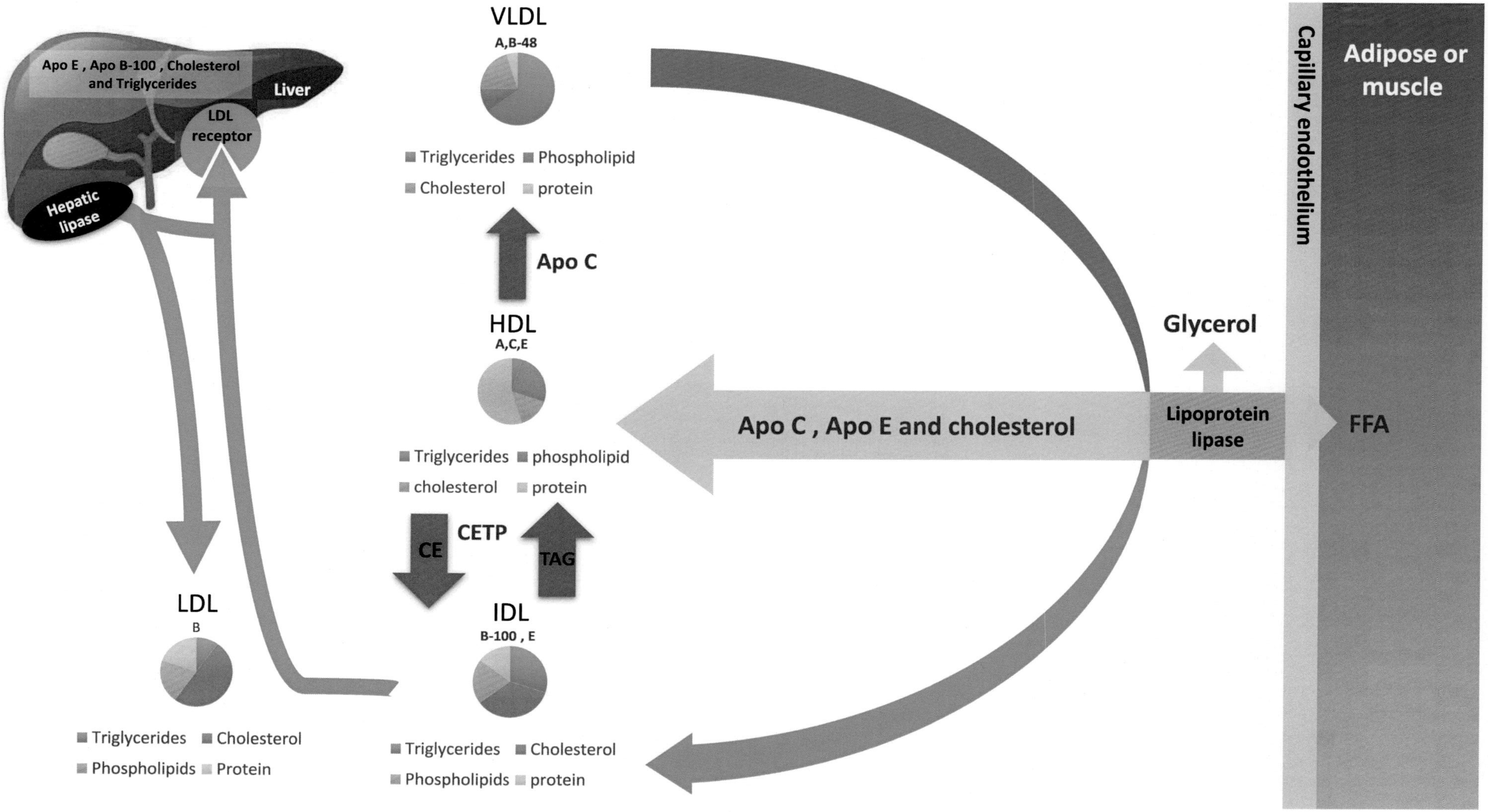
Apo E , Apo B-100 , Cholesterol and Triglycerides
Liver
LDL receptor
Hepatic lipase
VLDL
A,B-48
Triglycerides
Phospholipid
Cholesterol
protein
Apo C
HDL
A,C,E
Triglycerides
phospholipid
cholesterol
protein
CE
CETP
TAG
IDL
B-100 , E
Triglycerides
Cholesterol
Phospholipids
protein
LDL
B
Triglycerides
Cholesterol
Phospholipids
Protein
Apo C , Apo E and cholesterol
Lipoprotein lipase
Glycerol
Capillary endothelium
Adipose or muscle
FFA

Lipids, lipoproteins and cardiovascular disease

★ **High density Lipoproteins (HDL) or good cholesterol**

Smallest lipoproteins

Protective function against arterial disease

Synthesized in liver and intestinal

HDL metabolism

1. Nascent HDL synthesis in liver and gut acquires free cholesterol from extrahepatic cells, chylomicrons and VLDL, SO nasent HDL convert to HDL3

2. Cholesterol in HDL3 is esterified by the enzyme Lecithin cholesterol acytransferase (LCAT)

LCAT activated by apo A1

3. Then, cholesterol esters in HDL3 exchange with triglyceride in remnant chylomicrons and IDL by (CETP)

4. remnant chylomicrons and IDL removed from circulation by the liver, whence the cholesterol excreted in bile or bile acids

5. Much HDL2 recycled, but some removed from the circulation through scavenger receptor type B1 receptor (SRB1) in the liver

which recognize by apoA1 OR by hepatic triglyceride lipoprotein lipase (HTGL)

It contains the highest proportion of protein to lipids

functions

1. Source of apoproteins for chylomicrons and VLDL

2. Revers cholesterol transport, taking cholesterol from tissues to the liver

84

Lipids, lipoproteins and cardiovascular disease

HDL Metabolism

Lipids, lipoproteins and cardiovascular disease

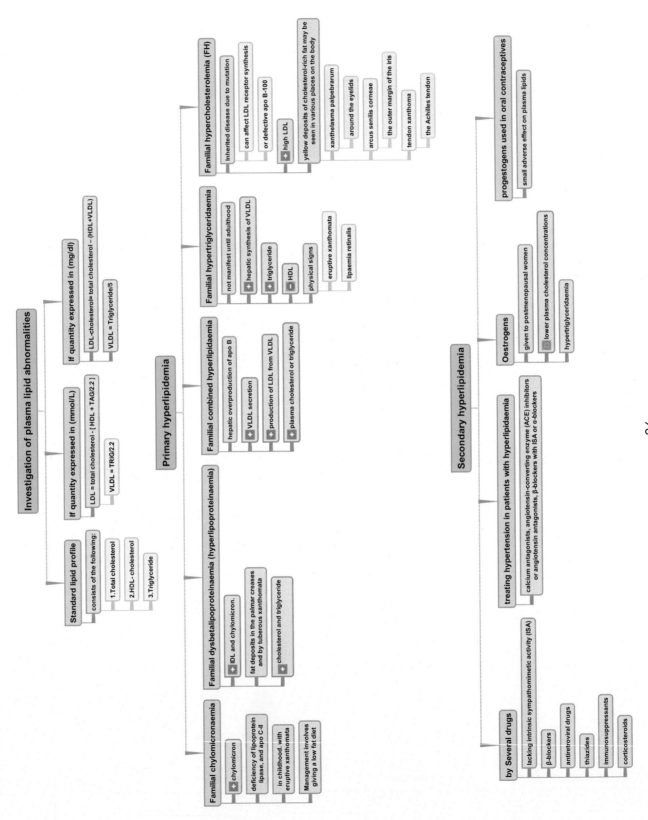

Investigation of plasma lipid abnormalities

Standard lipid profile
consists of the following:
- 1.Total cholesterol
- 2.HDL- cholesterol
- 3.Triglyceride

If quantity expressed in (mmol/L)
- LDL = total cholesterol - [HDL + TAG/2.2]
  - VLDL = TRIG/2.2

If quantity expressed in (mg/dl)
- LDL-cholesterol= total cholesterol – (HDL+VLDL)
  - VLDL = Triglyceride/5

Primary hyperlipidemia

Familial chylomicronaemia
- + chylomicron
- deficiency of lipoprotein lipase, and apo C-II
- in childhood, with eruptive xanthomata
- Management involves giving a low fat diet

Familial dysbetalipoproteinaemia (hyperlipoproteinaemia)
- + IDL and chylomicron.
- fat deposits in the palmar creases and by tuberous xanthomata
- + cholesterol and triglyceride

Familial combined hyperlipidaemia
- hepatic overproduction of apo B
- + VLDL secretion
- + production of LDL from VLDL
- + plasma cholesterol or triglyceride

Familial hypertriglyceridaemia
- not manifest until adulthood
- + hepatic synthesis of VLDL
- + triglyceride
- - HDL
- physical signs
  - eruptive xanthomata
  - lipaemia retinalis

Familial hypercholesterolemia (FH)
- Inherited disease due to mutation
- can affect LDL receptor synthesis or defective apo B-100
- + high LDL
- yellow deposits of cholesterol-rich fat may be seen in various places on the body
  - xanthelasma palpebrarum
  - around the eyelids
  - arcus senilis corneae
  - the outer margin of the iris
  - tendon xanthoma
  - the Achilles tendon

Secondary hyperlipidemia

treating hypertension in patients with hyperlipidaemia
- calcium antagonists, angiotensin-converting enzyme (ACE) inhibitors or angiotensin antagonists, β-blockers with ISA or α-blockers

by Several drugs
- lacking intrinsic sympathomimetic activity (ISA)
- β-blockers
- antiretroviral drugs
- thiazides
- immunosuppressants
- corticosteroids

Oestrogens
- given to postmenopausal women
- lower plasma cholesterol concentrations
- hypertriglyceridaemia

progestogens used in oral contraceptives
- small adverse effect on plasma lipids

Lipids, lipoproteins and cardiovascular disease

Atherosclerosis

Arteriosclerosis vs. atherosclerosis

Arteriosclerosis is the stiffening or hardening of the artery walls

Atherosclerosis is the narrowing of the artery because of plaque build-up. Atherosclerosis is a specific type of arteriosclerosis

All people with atherosclerosis have arteriosclerosis, but those with arteriosclerosis might not necessarily have atherosclerosis

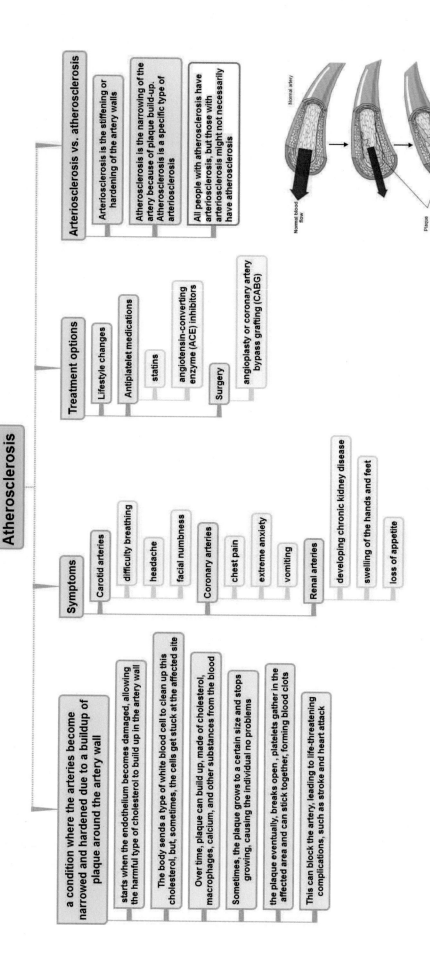

Treatment options

Lifestyle changes

Antiplatelet medications

statins

angiotensin-converting enzyme (ACE) inhibitors

Surgery

angioplasty or coronary artery bypass grafting (CABG)

Symptoms

Carotid arteries

difficulty breathing

headache

facial numbness

Coronary arteries

chest pain

extreme anxiety

vomiting

Renal arteries

developing chronic kidney disease

swelling of the hands and feet

loss of appetite

a condition where the arteries become narrowed and hardened due to a buildup of plaque around the artery wall

starts when the endothelium becomes damaged, allowing the harmful type of cholesterol to build up in the artery wall

The body sends a type of white blood cell to clean up this cholesterol, but, sometimes, the cells get stuck at the affected site

Over time, plaque can build up, made of cholesterol, macrophages, calcium, and other substances from the blood

Sometimes, the plaque grows to a certain size and stops growing, causing the individual no problems

the plaque eventually, breaks open , platelets gather in the affected area and can stick together, forming blood clots

This can block the artery, leading to life-threatening complications, such as stroke and heart attack

Stroke

A stroke occurs when the supply of blood to the brain is either interrupted or reduced

the brain does not get enough oxygen or nutrients, and brain cells start to die

Ischemic stroke

Hemorrhagic stroke

Hemorrhagic stroke

caused by blood leaking into the brain, so treatment focuses on controlling the bleeding and reducing the pressure on the brain

Treatment

begin with drugs given to reduce the pressure in the brain

prevent seizures and prevent sudden constrictions of blood vessels

Surgeons can place small clamps at the base of aneurysms or fill them with detachable coils to stop blood flow and prevent rupture

If the hemorrhage is caused by arteriovenous malformations (AVMs)

surgery can also be used to remove them if they are not too big and not too deep in the brain.

AVMs are tangled connections between arteries and veins that are weaker and burst more easily than other normal blood vessels

Ischemic stroke

caused by arteries being blocked or narrowed, and so treatment focuses on restoring an adequate flow of blood to the brain

Treatment

Injection of tissue plasminogen activator (TPA)

Aspirin

TPA is very effective at dissolving clots but needs to be injected within 4.5 hours of stroke symptoms starting

carotid endarterectomy involves a surgeon opening the carotid artery and removing any plaque that might be blocking it

angioplasty involves a surgeon inflating a small balloon in a narrowed artery via catheter and then inserting a mesh tube called a stent into the opening

This prevents the artery from narrowing again.

88

Endocrine hormones

you will organize your knowledge about :

The types of endocrine glands

The types of hormone and biochemical regulation

The types of endocrine control

The pitfalls in interpretation

The endocrine diseases

The anterior and posterior pituitary hormones

The regulation of thyroid hormone secretion

The thyroid function tests

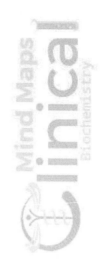

Endocrine hormones

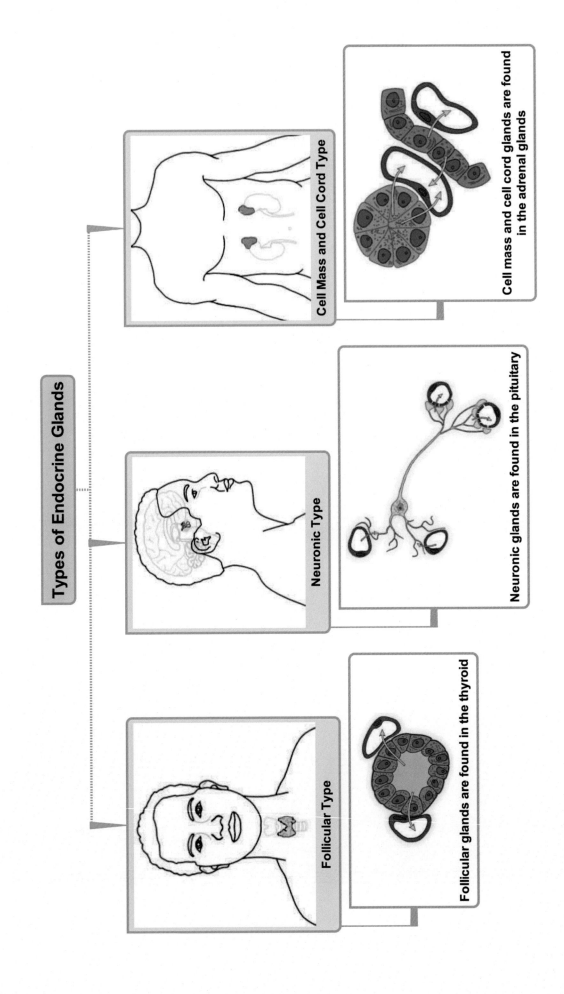

Types of Endocrine Glands

Follicular Type

Follicular glands are found in the thyroid

Neuronic Type

Neuronic glands are found in the pituitary

Cell Mass and Cell Cord Type

Cell mass and cell cord glands are found in the adrenal glands

90

Endocrine hormones

HORMONE ACTION

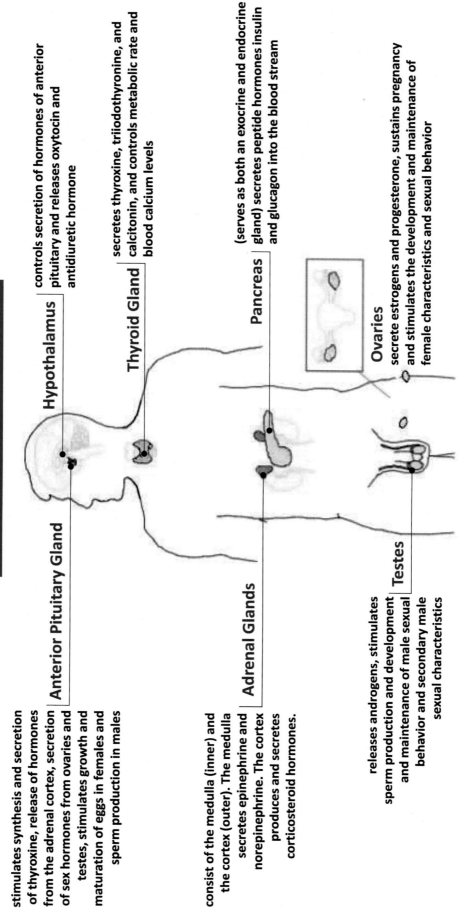

Hypothalamus — controls secretion of hormones of anterior pituitary and releases oxytocin and antidiuretic hormone

Anterior Pituitary Gland — stimulates synthesis and secretion of thyroxine, release of hormones from the adrenal cortex, secretion of sex hormones from ovaries and testes, stimulates growth and maturation of eggs in females and sperm production in males

Thyroid Gland — secretes thyroxine, triiodothyronine, and calcitonin, and controls metabolic rate and blood calcium levels

Pancreas — (serves as both an exocrine and endocrine gland) secretes peptide hormones insulin and glucagon into the blood stream

Adrenal Glands — consist of the medulla (inner) and the cortex (outer). The medulla secretes epinephrine and norepinephrine. The cortex produces and secretes corticosteroid hormones.

Ovaries — secrete estrogens and progesterone, sustains pregnancy and stimulates the development and maintenance of female characteristics and sexual behavior

Testes — releases androgens, stimulates sperm production and development and maintenance of male sexual behavior and secondary male sexual characteristics

91

HORMONES

chemical messenger that transport a signal from one cell to another
- Only a small amount of hormone is required to alter cell metabolism

affect only specific target tissues with specific receptors

Receptors constantly synthesized and broken down
- Down-regulation
- Up-regulation

Hormone structure
- Peptides or proteins
  - hypothalamic factor thyrotrophin-releasing hormone
    - has just 3 amino acids
  - pituitary gonadotrophins
    - large glycoproteins with subunits
- Amino acid derivatives
  - thyroid hormones
  - adrenaline
- Steroid hormones
  - glucocorticoids
  - sex steroid hormones
    - derived structurally from cholesterol

types of glands
- Exocrine – ducted
- Endocrine – ductless
  - (circulating hormones) – circulate in blood throughout body
  - Slower responses, effects last longer, broader influence

Assessment of endocrine control
- 1.Low concentrations
- 2.Variability
- 3.Hormone binding

Nervous system
- Neurotransmitters
- Faster responses, briefer effects, acts on specific target

92

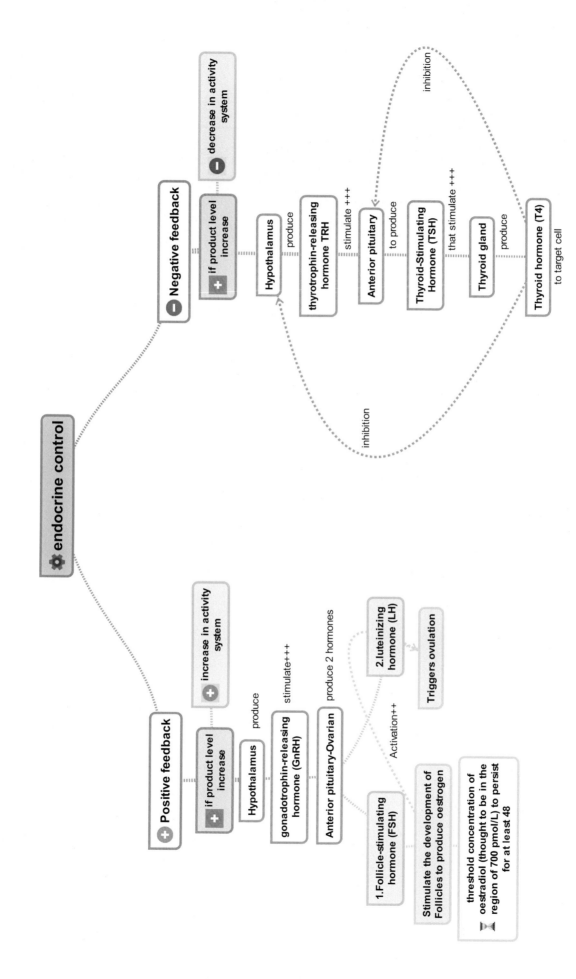

endocrine control

Positive feedback (+)

if product level increase (+)
→ increase in activity system (+)

Hypothalamus
produce

gonadotrophin-releasing hormone (GnRH)
stimulate+++

Anterior pituitary-Ovarian
produce 2 hormones

1.Follicle-stimulating hormone (FSH)
Stimulate the development of Follicles to produce oestrogen

⋈ threshold concentration of oestradiol (thought to be in the region of 700 pmol/L) to persist for at least 48

Activation++

2.luteinizing hormone (LH)
Triggers ovulation

Negative feedback (I)

if product level increase (+)
→ decrease in activity system (I)

Hypothalamus
produce

thyrotrophin-releasing hormone TRH
stimulate +++

Anterior pituitary
to produce

Thyroid-Stimulating Hormone (TSH)
that stimulate +++

Thyroid gland
produce

Thyroid hormone (T4)
to target cell

inhibition

inhibition

Endocrine hormones

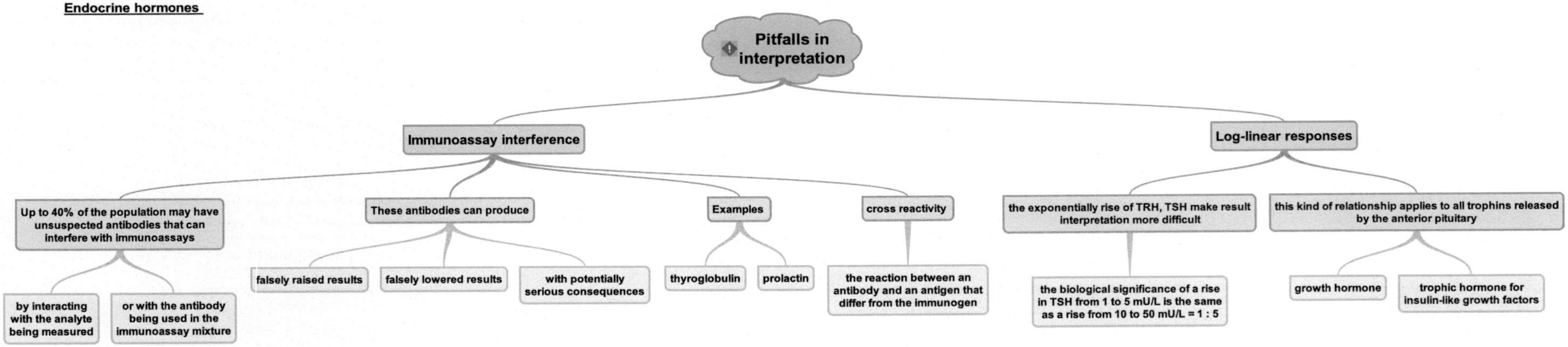

Pitfalls in interpretation

Log-linear responses

this kind of relationship applies to all trophins released by the anterior pituitary
- growth hormone
- trophic hormone for insulin-like growth factors

the exponentially rise of TRH, TSH make result interpretation more difficult
- the biological significance of a rise in TSH from 1 to 5 mU/L is the same as a rise from 10 to 50 mU/L = 1 : 5

Immunoassay interference

cross reactivity
- the reaction between an antibody and an antigen that differ from the immunogen

Examples
- thyroglobulin
- prolactin

These antibodies can produce
- falsely raised results
- falsely lowered results
- with potentially serious consequences

Up to 40% of the population may have unsuspected antibodies that can interfere with immunoassays
- by interacting with the analyte being measured
- or with the antibody being used in the immunoassay mixture

94

Endocrine hormones

Dynamic function tests

Insulin stress test (IST test)

- hypopituitarism is suspected
- used to diagnosis Cushing's disease
- Hypoglycemia: stimulus for ACTH release
- Assessment of anterior pituitary

| Hypothalamus |
| CRH |
| + Insulin |
| Anterior pituitary |
| ACTH |
| Adrenel cortex |
| Cortisol, GH & Aldosterone |

- + insulin
  - ⊖ glucose
  - Hypoglycemia
  - + ACTH
  - + GH
- Give Insulin after overnight fasting
  - to produce hypoglycaemic stress (blood glucose <2.2 mmol/L)
- Glucose level and Cortisol is measured every 30 min
  - This tests the ability of the anterior pituitary to produce ACTH and GH in response
- GH > 20 mU/L : NORMAL
- cortisol > 500 nmol/L: NORMAL

Thyrotrophin releasing hormone test (TRH test)

- To distinguish between hypothyroidism and hyperthyroidism
- used to assess the adequacy of anterior pituitary or hypothalamic disease

| Hypothalamus |
| TRH |
| + |
| Anterior pituitary |
| TSH |
| Thyroid |

- hypothyroidism
  - due to insufficient production of thyroid stimulating hormone (TSH)
  - caused by hypothalamic or pituitary defect
- ⊕ TSH
  - ⊕ T4
  - primary hypothyroidism
- ✕ TSH
  - defect in Anterior pituitary
  - Secondary hypothyroidism
- TRH is given as an intravenous bolus
  - blood sampling is at 0, 20, 60, 90 and 120 minutes
  - TSH >25 mU/L
    - ☀ hypothyroidism
  - TSH <2 mU/L
    - ☀ hyperthyroidism

Endocrine hormones

Pituitary responses to TRH

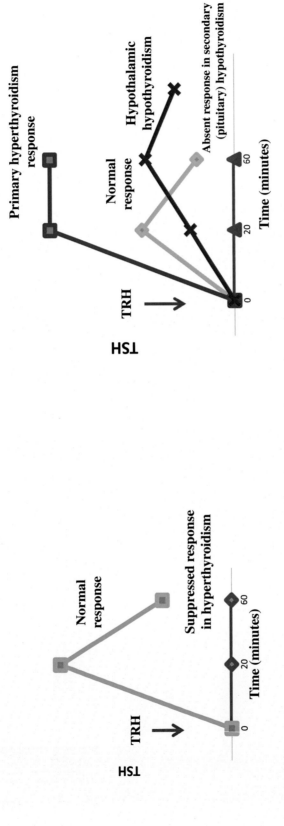

Used in investigation of pituitary or hypothalamic hypothyroidism

Used in investigation of hyperthyroidism

96

Endocrine hormones

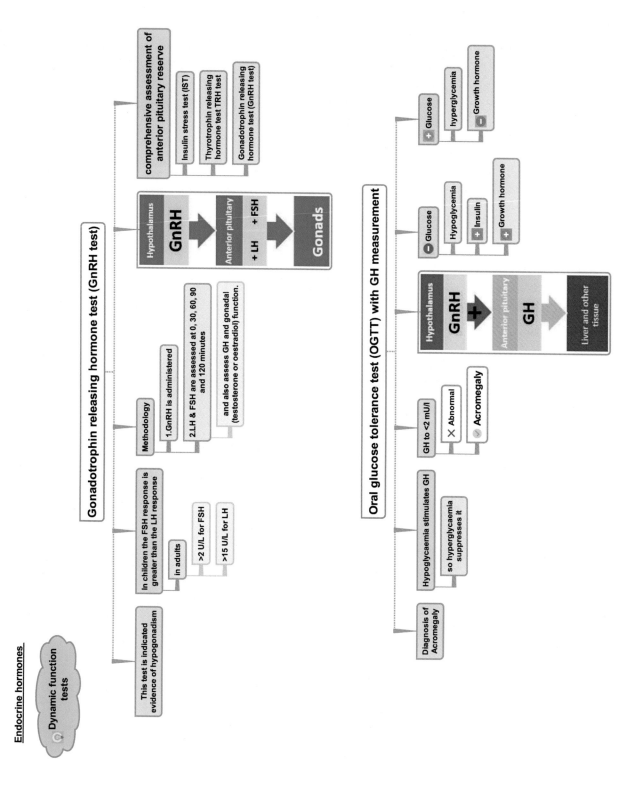

97

Endocrine hormones

Dynamic function tests

★ Synacthen tests

Short Synacthen test (SST)
- used to evaluate adrenal glucocorticoid secretion in response to synthetic ACTH (also known as tetracosactide or Synacthen)
- diagnosis of primary adrenal insufficiency
- Methodology:
  - two plasma cortisol samples have been taken after i.v. or i.m. administration of Synacthen 250 μg, one at 30 min and one at 60 min
  - ⊕ ACTH
  - ⊖ Cortisol
  - Primary adrenal insufficiency

- Short Synacthen test (SST) response
  - Basal sample > 225 nmol/L Cortisol
  - Final sample > 500 nmol/L Cortisol
  - Increment in cortisol at least = 200 nmol/L

Long Synacthen test
- Where the response to (SST) is inadequate or equivocal
- Methodology:
  - give Synacthen (1 mg) I.M for 3 days
  - normal response makes primary adrenal insufficiency unlikely (secondary adrenal insufficiency)
  - the SST repeated on the fourth (cortisol is measured at 0, 10, 30 and 60 minutes

Hypothalamus	CRH →
Anterior pituitary	ACTH →
Adrenal cortex	Cortisol

- ⊕ elevated ACTH in the presence of an impaired response to Synacthen
- primary adrenal failure

◎ Dexamethasone suppression tests

Low dose dexamethasone suppression test (1 mg)
- Methodology:
  - 1 mg dexamethasone orally at 23:00
  - cortisol blood test the following morning at 08:00 or 09:00
  - result, the cortisol has suppressed to <50 nmol/L

1 mg dexamethasone

Dexamethasone is an exogenous steroid that mimics the negative feedback of endogenous glucocorticoids

Hypothalamus	CRH →
Anterior pituitary	ACTH →
Adrenal cortex	Cortisol

High dose dexamethasone suppression test (8 mg)
- used to determine the source of elevated ACTH
  - ⊕ ACTH
    - pituitary (Cushing's disease)
      - ACTH production in Cushing's disease does usually suppress in response to high dose dexamethasone
    - ectopic ACTH production usually malignant
      - malignant production of ACTH usually does not

Assessment of hypothalamic-pituitary-adrenal axis

Endocrine hormones

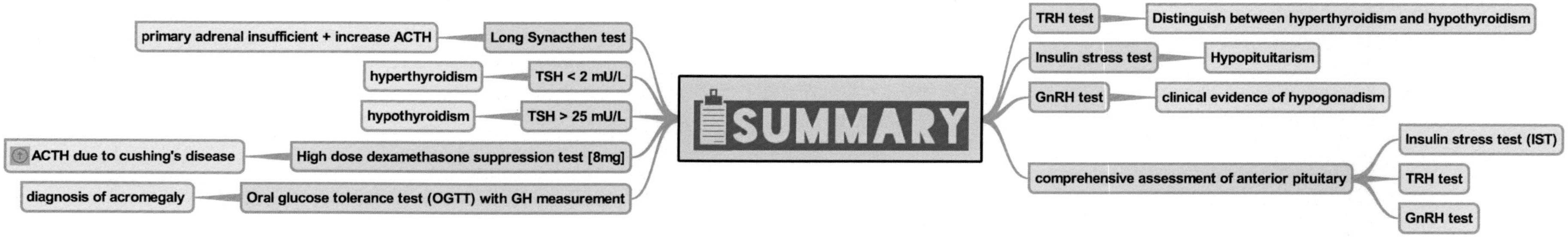

```
TRH test → Distinguish between hyperthyroidism and hypothyroidism
Insulin stress test → Hypopituitarism
GnRH test → clinical evidence of hypogonadism

Insulin stress test (IST)
TRH test          → comprehensive assessment of anterior pituitary
GnRH test
```

SUMMARY

```
primary adrenal insufficient + increase ACTH → Long Synacthen test
hyperthyroidism ← TSH < 2 mU/L
hypothyroidism ← TSH > 25 mU/L
ACTH due to cushing's disease ← High dose dexamethasone suppression test [8mg]
diagnosis of acromegaly ← Oral glucose tolerance test (OGTT) with GH measurement
```

Endocrine disease

Endocrine disease

Cushing's disease

- result of a pituitary adenoma
- secondary hypercortisolism
- (+) ACTH from the anterior pituitary
- Diagnosis by Insulin stress test (IST test) and measured the cortisol and GH

Acromegaly

- Due to pituitary adenoma
- (+) GH secretion
- Diagnosis by Oral glucose tolerance test (OGTT) with GH measurement

Addison's disease

- primary adrenal insufficiency and hypocortisolism
- the adrenal glands do not produce enough steroid hormones

Hypopituitarism

- Elderly patients may complain of symptoms relating to ACTH or TSH deficiency
  - hypoglycaemia
  - hypothermia
- Causes
  - infarction
  - congenital malformation
  - hypothalamic disorder
  - infection
  - tumor
  - trauma

Hyperprolactinaemia

- infertility in both sexes
  - women
    - amenorrhoea
    - galactorrhoea
  - men
    - large growing tumor begins to interfere with the optic nerves
- Causes
  - stress
  - seizures
  - primary hypothyroidism
  - idiopathic hypersecretion
  - prolactinoma

100

Pituitary function is regulated by the hypothalamus

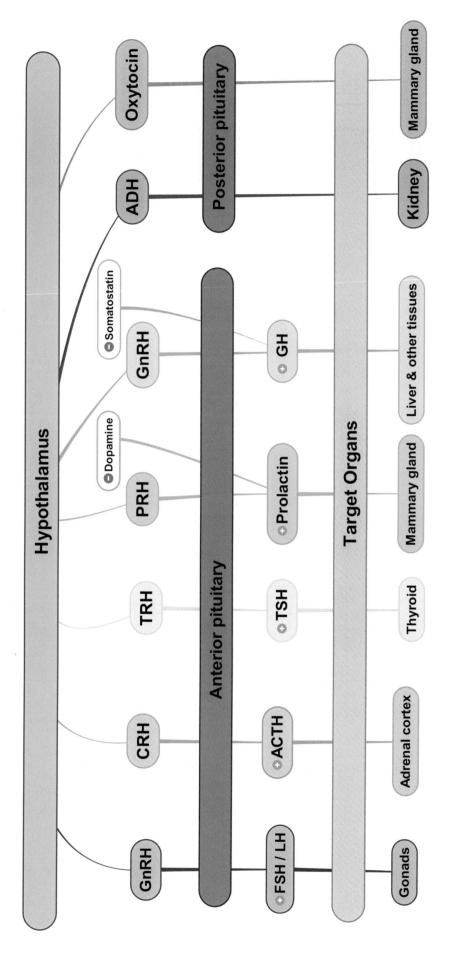

101

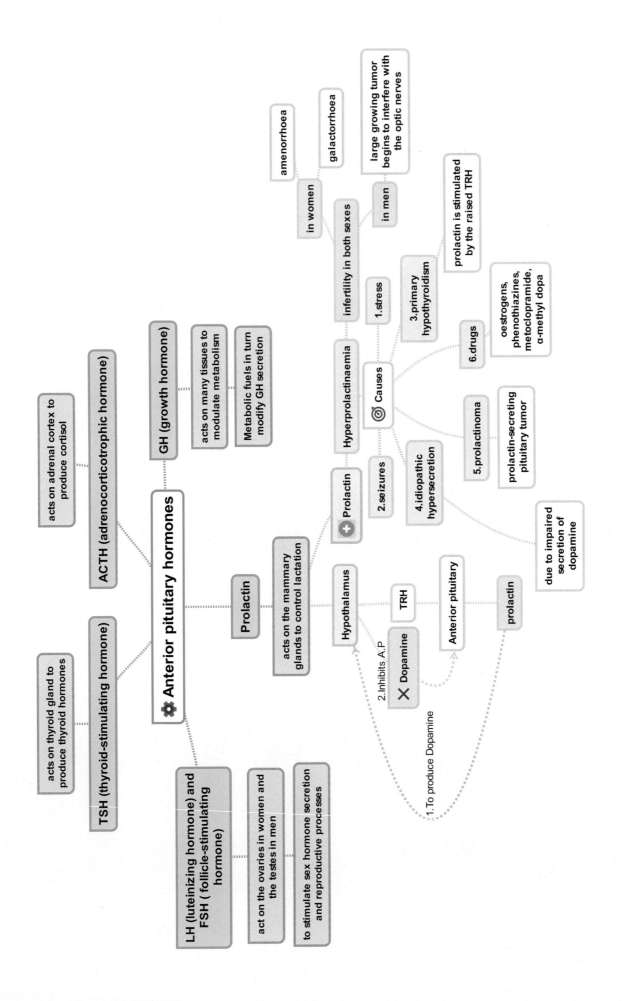

Anterior pituitary hormones

TSH (thyroid-stimulating hormone)
- acts on thyroid gland to produce thyroid hormones

ACTH (adrenocorticotrophic hormone)
- acts on adrenal cortex to produce cortisol

GH (growth hormone)
- acts on many tissues to modulate metabolism
- Metabolic fuels in turn modify GH secretion

Prolactin
- acts on the mammary glands to control lactation

LH (luteinizing hormone) and FSH (follicle-stimulating hormone)
- act on the ovaries in women and the testes in men
- to stimulate sex hormone secretion and reproductive processes

Hypothalamus
- TRH
- Dopamine
  - 1. To produce Dopamine
  - 2. Inhibits A.P
- Anterior pituitary
  - prolactin
    - due to impaired secretion of dopamine

Prolactin

Hyperprolactinaemia

infertility in both sexes
- in women
  - amenorrhoea
  - galactorrhoea
- in men
  - large growing tumor begins to interfere with the optic nerves

Causes
1. stress
2. seizures
3. primary hypothyroidism
   - prolactin is stimulated by the raised TRH
4. idiopathic hypersecretion
5. prolactinoma
   - prolactin-secreting pituitary tumor
6. drugs
   - oestrogens, phenothiazines, metoclopramide, α-methyl dopa

102

Endocrine hormones

Regulation of thyroid hormone secretion

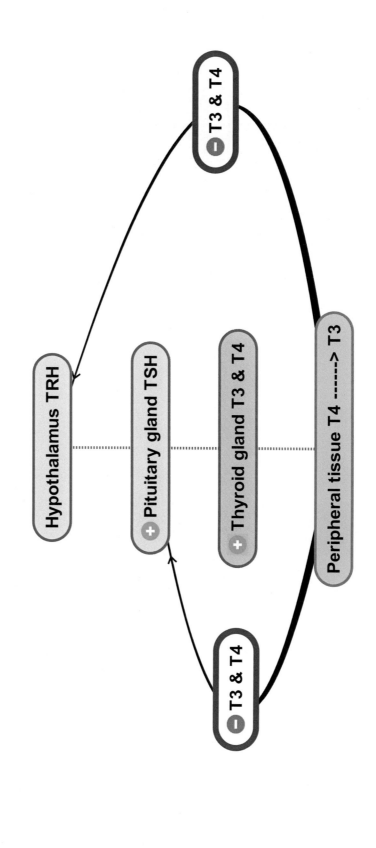

103

Endocrine hormones

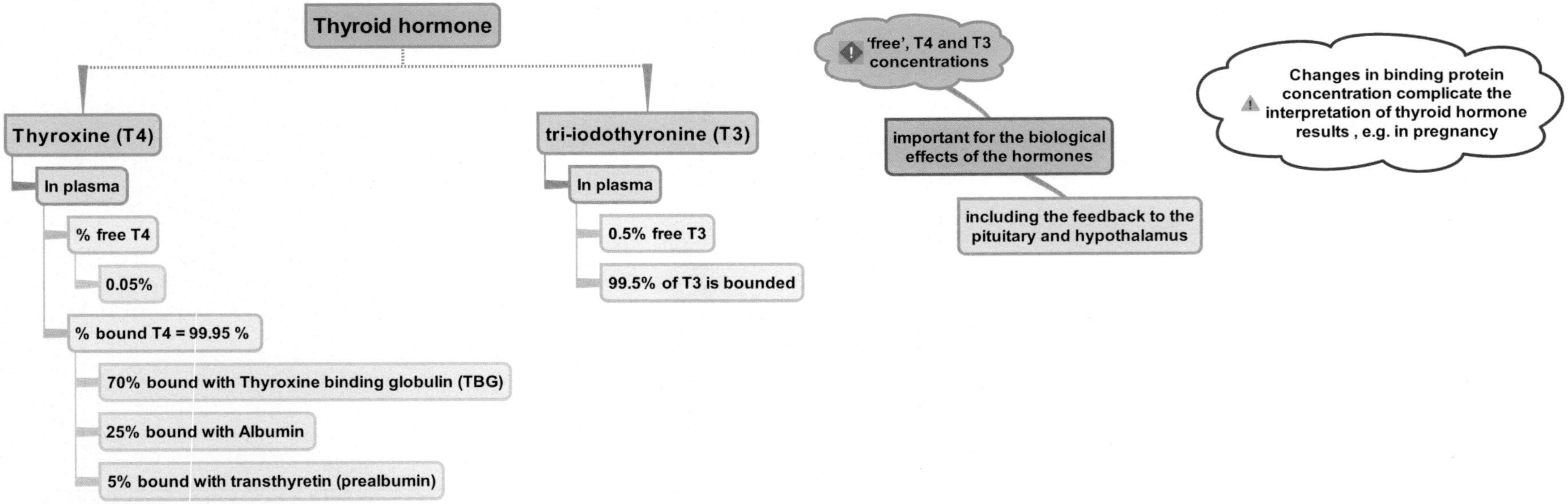

Thyroid hormone

Thyroxine (T4)

In plasma

% free T4

0.05%

% bound T4 = 99.95 %

70% bound with Thyroxine binding globulin (TBG)

25% bound with Albumin

5% bound with transthyretin (prealbumin)

tri-iodothyronine (T3)

In plasma

0.5% free T3

99.5% of T3 is bounded

'free', T4 and T3 concentrations

important for the biological effects of the hormones

including the feedback to the pituitary and hypothalamus

Changes in binding protein concentration complicate the interpretation of thyroid hormone results , e.g. in pregnancy

104

Endocrine hormones

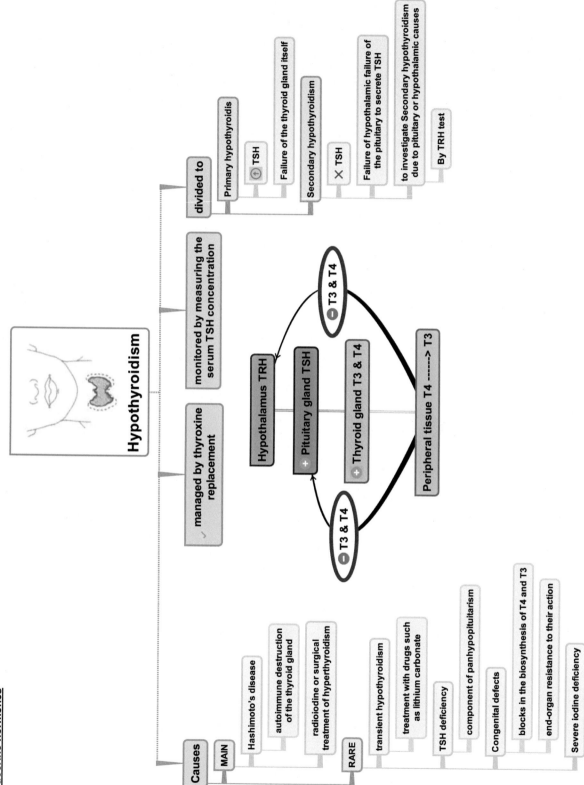

Hypothyroidism

- managed by thyroxine replacement
- monitored by measuring the serum TSH concentration
- divided to
  - Primary hypothyroidis
    - ↑ TSH
    - Failure of the thyroid gland itself
  - Secondary hypothyroidism
    - ✕ TSH
    - Failure of hypothalamic failure of the pituitary to secrete TSH
    - to investigate Secondary hypothyroidism due to pituitary or hypothalamic causes
    - By TRH test

Hypothalamus TRH
⊕ Pituitary gland TSH
⊕ Thyroid gland T3 & T4
Peripheral tissue T4 ------> T3

⊖ T3 & T4
⊖ T3 & T4

Causes

MAIN
- Hashimoto's disease
- autoimmune destruction of the thyroid gland
- radioiodine or surgical treatment of hyperthyroidism

RARE
- transient hypothyroidism
- treatment with drugs such as lithium carbonate
- TSH deficiency
- component of panhypopituitarism
- Congenital defects
- blocks in the biosynthesis of T4 and T3
- end-organ resistance to their action
- Severe iodine deficiency

105

Endocrine hormones

⚙ Strategy for the biochemical investigation of suspected hypothyroidism

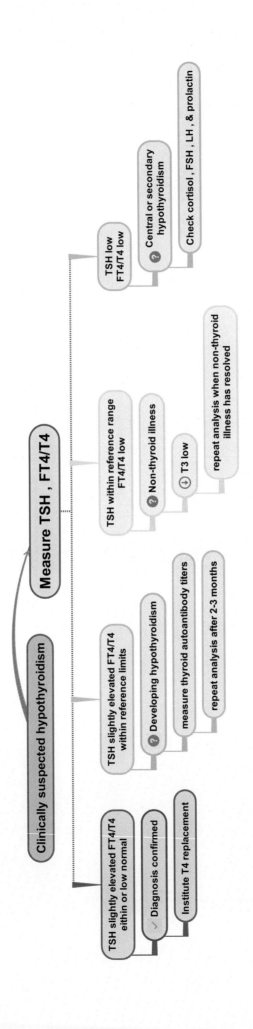

106

Endocrine hormones

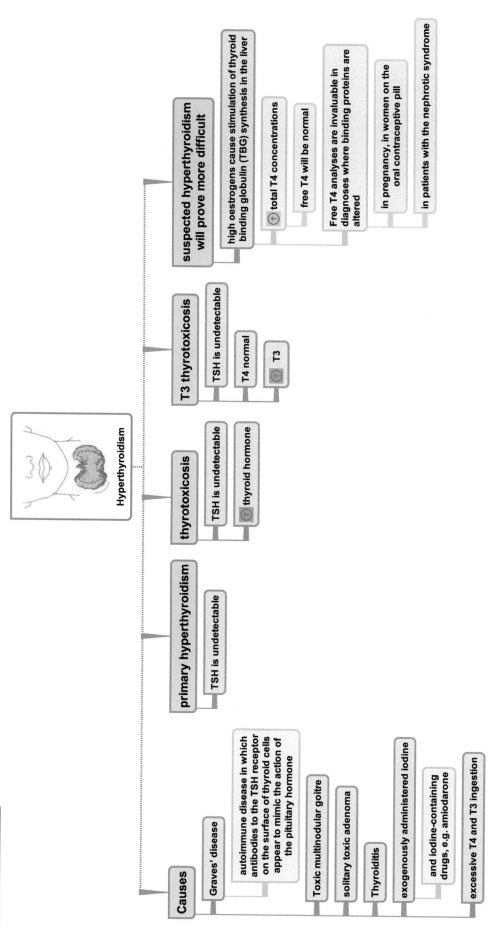

Hyperthyroidism

Causes
- Graves' disease
  - autoimmune disease in which antibodies to the TSH receptor on the surface of thyroid cells appear to mimic the action of the pituitary hormone
- Toxic multinodular goitre
- solitary toxic adenoma
- Thyroiditis
- exogenously administered iodine
- and iodine-containing drugs, e.g. amiodarone
- excessive T4 and T3 ingestion

primary hyperthyroidism
- TSH is undetectable

thyrotoxicosis
- TSH is undetectable
- ↑ thyroid hormone

T3 thyrotoxicosis
- TSH is undetectable
- T4 normal
- ↑ T3

suspected hyperthyroidism will prove more difficult
- high oestrogens cause stimulation of thyroid binding globulin (TBG) synthesis in the liver
  - ↑ total T4 concentrations
  - free T4 will be normal
- Free T4 analyses are invaluable in diagnoses where binding proteins are altered
  - in pregnancy, in women on the oral contraceptive pill
  - in patients with the nephrotic syndrome

Endocrine hormones

⚙ Strategy for the biochemical investigation of suspected Hyperthyroidism

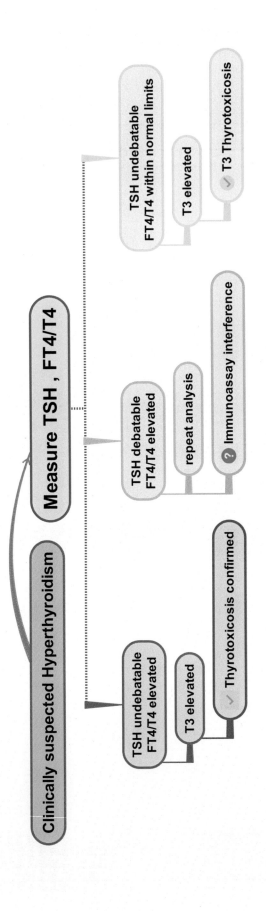

108

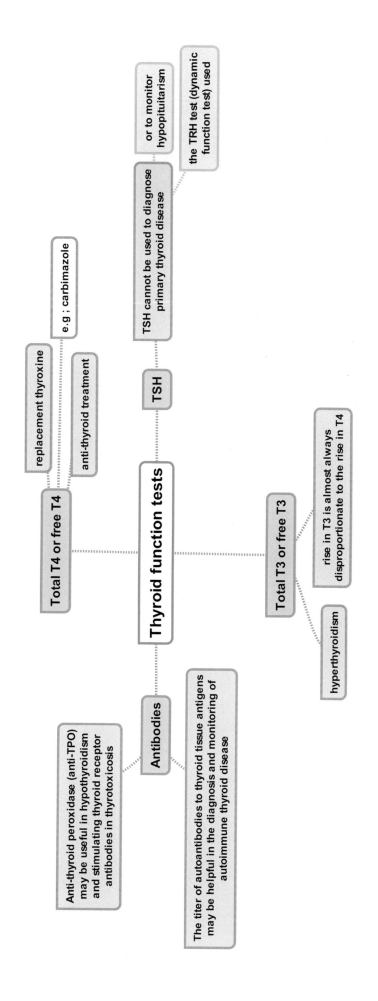

Thyroid function tests

Total T4 or free T4
- replacement thyroxine
- anti-thyroid treatment
  - e.g ; carbimazole

TSH
- TSH cannot be used to diagnose primary thyroid disease
  - or to monitor hypopituitarism
  - the TRH test (dynamic function test) used

Total T3 or free T3
- rise in T3 is almost always disproportionate to the rise in T4
- hyperthyroidism

Antibodies
- Anti-thyroid peroxidase (anti-TPO) may be useful in hypothyroidism and stimulating thyroid receptor antibodies in thyrotoxicosis
- The titer of autoantibodies to thyroid tissue antigens may be helpful in the diagnosis and monitoring of autoimmune thyroid disease

Drugs affecting thyroid function tests

Amiodarone

Mechanism
- Reduce peripheral deiodination
- stimulate or inhibit release of thyroid hormones from thyroid

Major effects
- ⊕ T4
- ⊝ T3
- ⊕ Transient TSH
- Hyperthyroidism
- hypothyroidism

Lithium

Mechanism
- Reduce thyroid uptake of iodine
- Reduce release of thyroid hormones from thyroid

Major effects
- Goitre
- hypothyroidism

Anticonvulsant (phenytoin , carbamazepine ,phenobarbital)

Mechanism
- Displace T4 & T3 from binding proteins

Major effects
- ⊕ free T4
- ⊕ free T3

Heparin

Mechanism
- Release LPL into plasma with resultant increase in free fatty acids
- these displace T4 & T3 from binding proteins

Major effects
- ⊕ free T4
- ⊕ free T3

Aspirin

Mechanism
- In high concentration , displaces T4 from transthyretin

Major effects
- ⊕ free T4

110

The cancer & tumor markers

you will organize your knowledge about :

The Benign and Malignant Tumor

The symptoms, stages, risk factors, causes, diagnosis and treatment for each type of cancer

The tumor markers

The Diagnostic Tests for Cancer

The Common tumor markers

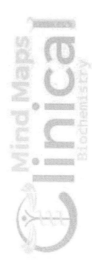

Mind Maps
Clinical
Biochemistry

111

The cancer & tumor markers

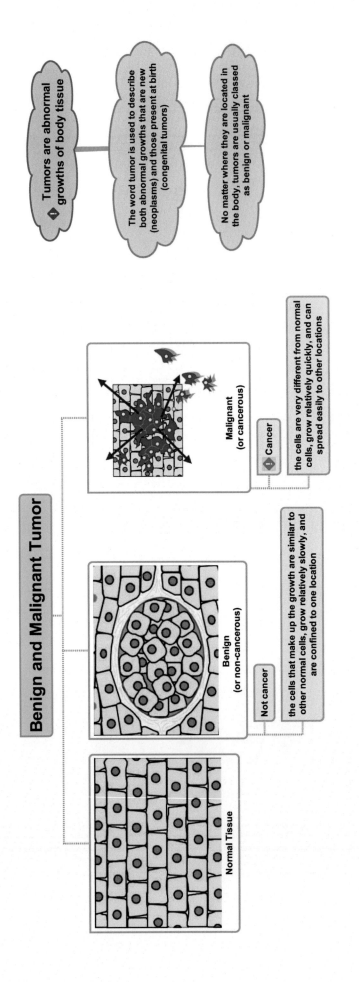

Tumors are abnormal growths of body tissue

The word tumor is used to describe both abnormal growths that are new (neoplasms) and those present at birth (congenital tumors)

No matter where they are located in the body, tumors are usually classed as benign or malignant

Benign and Malignant Tumor

Malignant (or cancerous)

◆ Cancer

the cells are very different from normal cells, grow relatively quickly, and can spread easily to other locations

Benign (or non-cancerous)

Not cancer

the cells that make up the growth are similar to other normal cells, grow relatively slowly, and are confined to one location

Normal Tissue

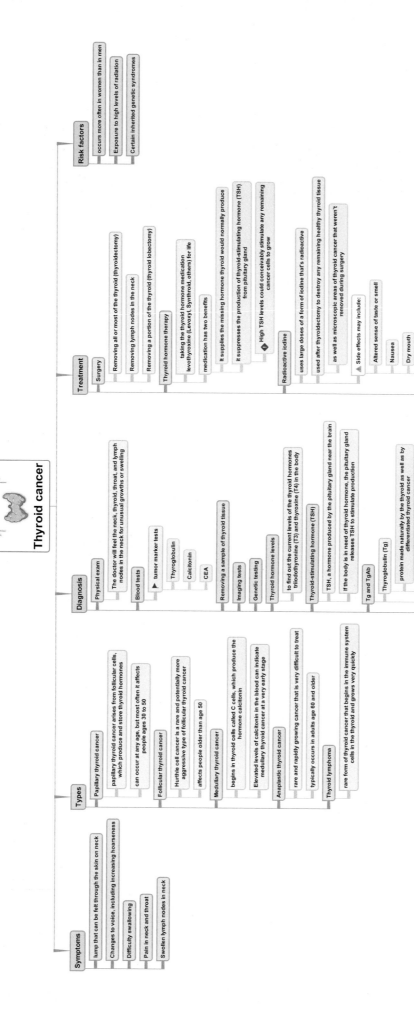

Thyroid cancer

Symptoms
- lump that can be felt through the skin on neck
- Changes to voice, including increasing hoarseness
- Difficulty swallowing
- Pain in neck and throat
- Swollen lymph nodes in neck

Types
- Papillary thyroid cancer
  - papillary thyroid cancer arises from follicular cells, which produce and store thyroid hormones
  - can occur at any age, but most often it affects people ages 30 to 50
- Follicular thyroid cancer
  - Hurthle cell cancer is a rare and potentially more aggressive type of follicular thyroid cancer
  - affects people older than age 50
- Medullary thyroid cancer
  - begins in thyroid cells called C cells, which produce the hormone calcitonin
  - Elevated levels of calcitonin in the blood can indicate medullary thyroid cancer at a very early stage
- Anaplastic thyroid cancer
  - rare and rapidly growing cancer that is very difficult to treat
  - typically occurs in adults age 60 and older
- Thyroid lymphoma
  - rare form of thyroid cancer that begins in the immune system cells in the thyroid and grows very quickly

Diagnosis
- Physical exam
  - The doctor will feel the neck, thyroid, throat, and lymph nodes in the neck for unusual growths or swelling
- Blood tests
  - tumor marker tests
    - Thyroglobulin
    - Calcitonin
    - CEA
- Removing a sample of thyroid tissue
- Imaging tests
- Genetic testing
- Thyroid hormone levels
  - to find out the current levels of the thyroid hormones triiodothyronine (T3) and thyroxine (T4) in the body
- Thyroid-stimulating hormone (TSH)
  - TSH, a hormone produced by the pituitary gland near the brain
  - If the body is in need of thyroid hormone, the pituitary gland releases TSH to stimulate production
- Tg and TgAb
  - Thyroglobulin (Tg)
    - protein made naturally by the thyroid as well as by differentiated thyroid cancer
    - After treatment, there should be very low levels of thyroglobulin in the blood
    - If Tg is rising after surgery and/or radioactive iodine, it may be a sign of more cancer
  - test for thyroglobulin antibodies (TgAb)
    - are proteins produced by the body to attack thyroglobulin that occur in some patients
    - If TgAb is found, it is known to interfere with the results of the Tg level test
- Medullary type-specific tests
  - check for high calcitonin and carcinoembryonic antigen (CEA) levels
  - blood test to detect the presence of RET proto-oncogenes

Treatment
- Surgery
  - Removing all or most of the thyroid (thyroidectomy)
  - Removing lymph nodes in the neck
  - Removing a portion of the thyroid (thyroid lobectomy)
- Thyroid hormone therapy
  - taking the thyroid hormone medication levothyroxine (Levoxyl, Synthroid, others) for life
  - medication has two benefits
    - It supplies the missing hormone thyroid would normally produce
    - It suppresses the production of thyroid-stimulating hormone (TSH) from pituitary gland
      - High TSH levels could conceivably stimulate any remaining cancer cells to grow
- Radioactive iodine
  - uses large doses of a form of iodine that's radioactive
  - used after thyroidectomy to destroy any remaining healthy thyroid tissue as well as microscopic areas of thyroid cancer that weren't removed during surgery
  - Side effects may include:
    - Altered sense of taste or smell
    - Nausea
    - Dry mouth
    - Dry eyes
- External radiation therapy
- Chemotherapy
- Targeted drug therapy
  - Vandetanib (Caprelsa)
  - Cabozantinib (Cometriq)
  - Sorafenib (Nexavar)

Risk factors
- occurs more often in women than in men
- Exposure to high levels of radiation
- Certain inherited genetic syndromes

113

The cancer & tumor markers

Prostate cancer

Symptoms
- frequent urges to urinate, including at night
- difficulty commencing and maintaining urination
- blood in the urine
- painful urination and, less commonly, ejaculation
- difficulty achieving or maintaining an erection may be difficult
- bone pain, often in the spine, femur, pelvis, or ribs

Diagnosis
- digital rectal examination (DRE)
- biomarker test checking the blood, urine, or body tissues
- PCA3 test examining the urine for the PCA3 gene only found in prostate cancer cells
- transrectal ultrasound scan providing imaging of the affected region using a probe that emits sounds
- biopsy, or the removal of 12 to 14 small pieces of tissue from several areas of the prostate for examination under a microscope
- bone, CT scan, or MRI scan
- Clinical tumor marker
- prostate-specific antigen (PSA)

Treatment
- Early stage prostate cancer
  - Watchful waiting or monitoring
  - PSA blood levels are regularly checked
- Radical prostatectomy
  - The prostate is surgically removed
- Brachytherapy
  - Radioactive seeds are implanted into the prostate to deliver targeted radiation treatment
- Conformal radiation therapy
  - Radiation beams are shaped so that the region where they overlap is as close to the same shape as the organ or region that requires treatment
  - This minimizes healthy tissue exposure to radiation
- Intensity modulated radiation therapy
- Advanced prostate cancer
  - Chemotherapy
  - Androgen deprivation therapy (ADT)
    - is a hormone treatment that reduces the effect of androgen
    - Androgens are male hormones that can stimulate cancer growth.
    - ADT can slow down and even stop cancer growth by reducing androgen levels
    - The patient will likely need long-term hormone therapy.

Risk factors
- Age
  - rare among men under the age of 45 years
  - more common after the age of 50 years
- Geography
  - occurs most frequently in North America, northwestern Europe, on the Caribbean islands, and in Australia
- Genetic factors
- Diet
  - a diet high in red meat or high-fat dairy products may increase a person's chances of developing prostate cancer
- Medication
  - non-steroidal anti-inflammatory drug (NSAID)
  - reduce the risk of prostate cancer
- Obesity
  - obesity is linked to the development of prostate cancer
- Agent Orange

prevention
- Maintain a healthy weight
- Exercise most days of the week
- Choose a healthy diet
- Choose a low-fat diet
- Eat more fat from plants than from animals
- Increase the amount of fruits and vegetables you eat each day
- Eat fish
- Reduce the amount of dairy products you eat each day

114

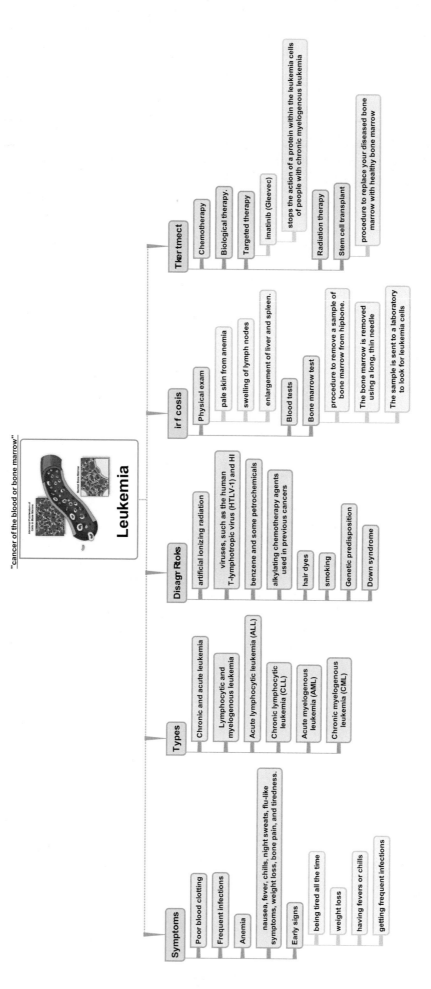

"cancer of the blood or bone marrow"

Leukemia

Symptoms
- Poor blood clotting
- Frequent infections
- Anemia
- nausea, fever, chills, night sweats, flu-like symptoms, weight loss, bone pain, and tiredness.
- Early signs
  - being tired all the time
  - weight loss
  - having fevers or chills
  - getting frequent infections

Types
- Chronic and acute leukemia
- Lymphocytic and myelogenous leukemia
- Acute lymphocytic leukemia (ALL)
- Chronic lymphocytic leukemia (CLL)
- Acute myelogenous leukemia (AML)
- Chronic myelogenous leukemia (CML)

Disease Risks
- artificial ionizing radiation
- viruses, such as the human T-lymphotropic virus (HTLV-1) and HI
- benzene and some petrochemicals
- alkylating chemotherapy agents used in previous cancers
- hair dyes
- smoking
- Genetic predisposition
- Down syndrome

Diagnosis
- Physical exam
  - pale skin from anemia
  - swelling of lymph nodes
  - enlargement of liver and spleen.
- Blood tests
- Bone marrow test
  - procedure to remove a sample of bone marrow from hipbone.
  - The bone marrow is removed using a long, thin needle
  - The sample is sent to a laboratory to look for leukemia cells

Treatment
- Chemotherapy
- Biological therapy.
- Targeted therapy
  - imatinib (Gleevec)
  - stops the action of a protein within the leukemia cells of people with chronic myelogenous leukemia
- Radiation therapy
- Stem cell transplant
  - procedure to replace your diseased bone marrow with healthy bone marrow

115

The cancer & tumor markers

Bone Marrow Biopsy

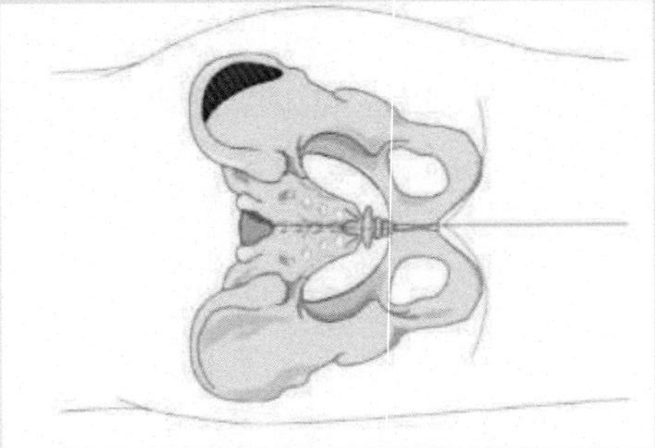

Posterior view of pelvic region with target area for bone marrow biopsy highlighted.

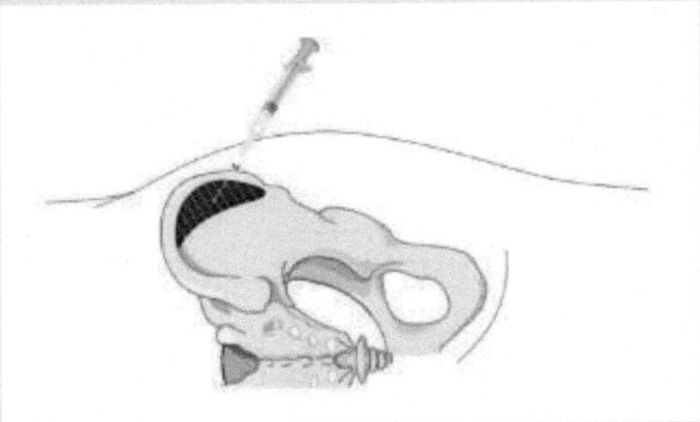

Posterior view of pelvis with hypodermic needle penetrating skin at an angle to reach the ilium just below the iliac crest

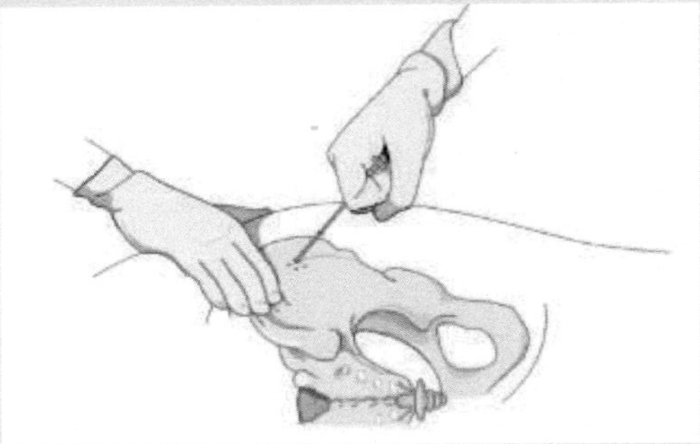

Procedure used to obtain a bone marrow sample for biopsy from the ilium by aspiration through a needle

116

Non-Hodgkin's lymphoma

Lymphatic System

Symptoms

- Painless, swollen lymph nodes in your neck, armpits or groin
- Abdominal pain or swelling
- Chest pain, coughing or trouble breathing
- Persistent fatigue
- Fever
- Night sweats
- Unexplained weight loss

TeDlagntors

- Medications that suppress immune system
- Infection with certain viruses and bacteria
- Certain chemicals, such as those used to kill insects and weeds
- the risk increases with age
- In people 60 or over

Rypks

- Chronic lymphocytic leukemia
  - type of cancer of the blood and bone marrow — the spongy tissue inside bones where blood cells are made
- Cutaneous B-cell lymphoma
  - a rare type of cancer that begins in the white blood cells and attacks the skin
  - begins in the B cells — one type of disease-fighting white blood cells called lymphocytes
- Cutaneous T-cell lymphoma
  - a rare type of cancer that begins in the white blood cells and attacks the skin.
  - is one of several types of lymphoma collectively called non-Hodgkin lymphoma
- Follicular lymphoma
  - type of non-Hodgkin lymphoma (NHL). It develops when the body makes abnormal B-cells — the lymphoma cells
- Waldenstrom macroglobulinemia
  - bone marrow produces too many abnormal white blood cells that crowd out healthy blood cells
  - The abnormal white blood cells produce a protein that accumulates in the blood, impairs circulation and causes complications

Stg ksi

- Stage I
  - Cancer has limited to one lymph node region or a group of nearby nodes
- Stage II
  - the cancer has invaded one organ and the nearby lymph nodes
- Stage III
  - found in the lymph nodes above the diaphragm and in the spleen
- Stage IV
  - affect other parts of the body, such as the liver, lungs or bones.

f g cosss

- Physical exam
  - check for swollen lymph nodes, including in neck, underarm and groin, as well as for a swollen spleen or liver
- Lymph node test
  - lymph node biopsy procedure to remove all or part of a lymph node for laboratory testing
- Imaging tests
  - computerized tomography (CT)
  - positron emission tomography (PET)
- Blood and urine tests
- Bone marrow test
  - inserting a needle into hipbone to remove a sample of bone marrow
  - The sample is analyzed to look for non-Hodgkin's lymphoma cells

Rrkgtfmkct

- Chemotherapy
- Targeted therapy
- Biological therapy
- Bone marrow transplant
  - treat Waldenstrom macroglobulinemia
  - high doses of chemotherapy are used to wipe out diseased bone marrow
  - Healthy blood stem cells are infused into body where they can rebuild healthy bone marrow
- Other drug therapy
  - rituximab (Rituxan)
    - type of monoclonal antibody that attaches to B cells and makes them more visible to the immune system, which can then attack
  - Ibrutinib (Imbruvica)

117

NON-HODGKIN LYMPHOMA

Non-Hodgkin lymphoma is cancer that begins in cells of the immune system. The immune system fights infections and other diseases.

Because lymphatic tissue is in many parts of the body, Hodgkin lymphoma can start almost anywhere. Usually, it's first found in a lymph node.

The lymphatic system is part of the immune system:

Lymph nodes:

Lymph vessels are connected to small, round masses of tissue called lymph nodes. Groups of lymph nodes are found in the neck, underarms, chest, abdomen, and groin. Lymph nodes store white blood cells. They trap and remove bacteria or other harmful substances that may be in the lymph.

Other parts of the lymphatic system:

Other parts of the lymphatic system: Other parts of the lymphatic system include the tonsils, thymus, and spleen. Lymphatic tissue is also found in other parts of the body including the stomach, skin, and small intestine.

Lymph vessels:

The lymphatic system has a network of lymph vessels. Lymph vessels branch into all the tissues of the body

Lymph:

The lymph vessels carry clear fluid called lymph. Lymph contains white blood cells, especially lymphocytes such as B cells and T cells.

118

The cancer & tumor markers

Breast cancer

Symptoms
- pain in the armpit or breast that does not change with the monthly cycle
- pitting or redness of the skin of the breast, like the skin of an orange
- a rash around or on one of the nipples
- discharge from a nipple, possibly containing blood
- a sunken or inverted nipple
- peeling, flaking, or scaling of the skin on the breast or nipple

Stages
- **Stage 0** – Known as ductal carcinoma in situ (DCIS), the cells are limited to within a duct and have not invaded surrounding tissues.
- **Stage 1** – the tumor is up to 2 centimeters (cm) across and it has not affected any lymph nodes.
- **Stage 2** – the tumor is 2 cm across and it has started to spread to nearby nodes.
- **Stage 3** – the tumor is up to 5 cm across and it may have spread to some lymph nodes.
- **Stage 4** – the cancer has spread to distant organs, especially the bones, liver, brain, or lungs.

Risk factors
- **Age** – As 20 years, the chance of developing breast cancer in the next decade is 0.6 percent. By the age of 70 years, this figure goes up to 3.8 percent.
- **Genetics** – If a woman carries the BRCA1 and BRCA2 genes have a higher risk of developing breast cancer, ovarian cancer, or both. Women who carry the BRCA1 and BRCA2 genes have a higher risk of developing breast cancer. These genes can be inherited. These genes are also linked to a greater breast cancer risk.
- **A history of breast cancer or breast lumps** – Women who have had breast cancer before are more likely to have it again, compared with those who have no history of the disease. Having some types of benign, or non-cancerous breast lumps increases the chance of developing cancer later on. Examples include atypical ductal hyperplasia or lobular carcinoma in situ.
- **Dense breast tissue** – develop in higher density breast tissue
- **Estrogen exposure and breastfeeding** – Being exposed to estrogen for a longer period appears to increase the risk of breast cancer. This could be due to starting periods earlier or entering menopause later than average. Between these times, estrogen levels are higher. Breastfeeding, especially for over 1 year, appears to reduce the chance of developing breast cancer.
- **Body weight** – Women who are overweight or have obesity after menopause may have a higher risk of developing breast cancer, due to higher levels of estrogen. High sugar intake may also be a factor.
- **Alcohol consumption** – Women who consume more than 3 drinks a day have a 1.5 times higher risk.
- **Hormone treatments** – The use of hormone replacement therapy (HRT) and oral birth control pills have been linked to breast cancer.
- **Radiation exposure** – Undergoing radiation treatment for a cancer that is not breast cancer increases the risk of breast cancer later in life.
- **Occupational hazards** – In 2012, researchers concluded that exposure to certain carcinogens and endocrine disruptors, for example in the workplace, could be linked to breast cancer. In 2007, scientists suggested that working night shifts could increase the risk of breast cancer, but more recent research concludes that is unlikely.

Causes
- After puberty, a woman's breast consists of fat, connective tissue, and thousands of lobules, tiny glands that produce milk for breastfeeding.
- ...ducts, carry the milk toward the nipple
- In cancer, the body's cells multiply uncontrollably. It is the excessive cell growth that causes cancer.
- Breast cancer usually starts in the inner lining of milk ducts or the lobules that supply them with milk.
- From there, it can spread to other parts of the body.

Types
- **Ductal carcinoma** – This begins in the milk duct and is the most common type.
- **Lobular carcinoma** – This starts in the lobules.
- **Invasive breast cancer** – when the cancer cells break out from inside the lobules or ducts and invade nearby tissue.
- **Non-invasive breast cancer** – when the cancer is still within its place of origin and has not broken out. These cells can eventually develop into invasive breast cancer.
- Breast cancer can also affect men, but it is less common in men than in women.

Diagnosis
- **Breast exam** – The physician will check the patient's breasts for lumps and other symptoms. The patient will be asked to sit or stand with their arms in different positions, such as above the head and by her sides.
- **Imaging tests**
  - mammogram – type of x-ray commonly used for initial breast cancer screening
  - ultrasound scan – A produces images that can help differentiate between a solid mass or a fluid-filled cyst
  - MRI scan – involves injecting a dye into the patient, so find out how far the cancer has spread
- **Biopsy** – A sample of tissue is surgically removed for laboratory analysis. This can show whether the cells are cancerous, and, if so, which type of cancer it is, including whether or not the cancer is hormone-sensitive.
- **Clinical tumor markers**
  - CA 15-3
  - CA 27-29
  - CEA
- Diagnosis also involves **staging the cancer**, to establish:
  - the size of a tumor
  - ow far it has spread
  - whether it is invasive or non-invasive
  - whether it has metastasized, or spread to other parts of the body

Treatment
- **Surgery**
  - **Lumpectomy** – Removing the tumor and a small margin of healthy tissue around it can help prevent the spread of the cancer. This may be an option if the tumor is small and likely to be easy to separate from the surrounding tissue.
  - **Mastectomy** – Simple mastectomy involves removing the lobules, ducts, fatty tissue, nipple, areola, and some skin. Radical mastectomy removes muscle from the chest wall and the lymph nodes in the armpit as well.
  - **Sentinel node biopsy** – Removing one lymph node can stop the cancer spreading. If breast cancer reaches a lymph node, it can spread further through the lymphatic system into other parts of the body.
  - **Axillary lymph node dissection** – If there are cancer cells on a node called the sentinel node, the surgeon may recommend removing several lymph nodes in the armpit to prevent the spread of disease.
  - **Reconstruction** – Following breast surgery, reconstruction can increase the breast so that it looks similar to the other breast. This can be done at the same time as a mastectomy, or at a later date.
- **Radiation therapy** – Used from around a month after surgery. It can kill any remaining cancer cells. Each session lasts a few minutes, and the patient may need three to five sessions per week for 3 to 6 weeks.
  - **Adverse effects** – Fatigue, lymphedema, darkening of the breast skin, and irritation of the breast skin.
- **Chemotherapy** – **adjuvant chemotherapy** – Medication known as cytotoxic drugs may be used to kill cancer cells, if there is a high risk of recurrence or spread. **neo-adjuvant chemotherapy** – If the tumor is large, chemotherapy may be administered before surgery to shrink the tumor and make its removal easier.
  - **Adverse effects** – nausea, vomiting, loss of appetite, fatigue, sore mouth, hair loss, and a slightly higher susceptibility to infections.
- **Hormone blocking therapy** – Used to prevent recurrence in hormone-sensitive breast cancers, referred to as estrogen receptor (ER) positive and progesterone receptor (PR) positive cancers. Hormone blocking therapy is normally used after surgery, but it may sometimes be used beforehand to shrink the tumor. It may be the only option for patients who cannot undergo surgery, chemotherapy, or radiotherapy. This effects can normally last for up to 5 years after surgery.
  - **Examples**
    - tamoxifen
    - aromatase inhibitors
    - ovarian ablation or suppression
    - a luteinizing hormone-releasing hormone agonist (LHRH) drug called Goserelin, in suppresses the ovaries
- **Biological treatment** – Targeted drugs destroy specific types of breast cancer.
  - trastuzumab (Herceptin)
  - lapatinib (Tykerb)
  - bevacizumab (Avastin)

Prevention
There is no sure way to prevent breast cancer, but some lifestyle decisions can significantly reduce the risk of breast and other types of cancer.
- avoiding excess alcohol consumption
- healthy diet with plenty of fresh fruit and vegetables
- getting enough exercise
- maintaining a healthy body mass index (BMI)
- Preventive surgery is an option for women at high risk

Bladder cancer

Symptoms
- Blood in urine (hematuria)
- Painful urination
- Pelvic pain
- Back pain
- Frequent urination

But, these symptoms often occur because of something other than bladder cancer

gesRa
- Smoking
- Exposure to chemicals
- Past radiation exposure
- Chronic irritation of the lining of the bladder
- Parasitic infections

lypRe
- Urothelial carcinoma — occurs in the cells that line the inside of the bladder
- Squamous cell carcinoma — associated with chronic irritation of the bladder
- Adenocarcinoma — occurs in cells that make up mucus-secreting glands in the bladder

k sf orgZtoua
- Smoking
- Increasing age — rarely found in people younger than 40
- Being white
- Being a man — Men are more likely to develop bladder cancer than women are
- Exposure to certain chemicals — arsenic and chemicals used in the manufacture of dyes, rubber, leather, textiles and paint products
- Previous cancer treatment — Treatment with the anti-cancer drug cyclophosphamide increases the risk of bladder cancer
- Chronic bladder inflammation — Increase the risk of a squamous cell bladder cancer
- Personal or family history of cancer — A family history of hereditary nonpolyposis colorectal cancer, also called Lynch syndrome, can increase the risk of cancer in the urinary system

T gDhoss
- Cystoscopy
- Biopsy
- Urine cytology
- Imaging tests
- Determining the extent of the cancer — To determine whether cancer has spread to lymph nodes or to other areas of body
  - CT scan
  - Magnetic resonance imaging (MRI)
  - Bone scan
  - Chest X-ray
- Clinical tumor marker
  - CYFRA 21-1
  - Bladder tumor antigens (BTA)
  - Nuclear matrix proteins (NMP-22)
  - Nuclear matrix proteins (NMP-52)

i RgtmRnt
- Surgery — remove cancerous tissue
- Transurethral resection of bladder tumor (TURBT)
- Cystectomy
- Neobladder reconstruction
- Ileal conduit
- Continent urinary reservoir
- Chemotherapy in the bladder (intravesical chemotherapy) — to treat tumors that are confined to the lining of the bladder but have a high risk of recurrence or progression to a higher stage
- Reconstruction — to create a new way for urine to exit the body after bladder removal
- Chemotherapy for the whole body (systemic chemotherapy) — to increase the chance for a cure in a person having surgery to remove the bladder / or as a primary treatment in cases where surgery isn't an option
- Radiation therapy — to destroy cancer cells, often as a primary treatment in cases where surgery isn't an option or isn't desired
- Immunotherapy — to trigger the body's immune system to fight cancer cells, either in the bladder or throughout the body

PuRvRnt on
- Don't smoke
- Take caution around chemicals
- The antioxidants in fruits and vegetables may help reduce risk of cancer

Male Urinary Tract

Female Urinary Tract

120

Colorectal cancer

Symptoms
- changes in bowel habits
- diarrhea or constipation
- feeling that the bowel does not empty properly after a bowel movement
- blood in feces that makes stools look black
- bright red blood coming from the rectum
- pain and bloating in the abdomen
- feeling of fullness in the abdomen, even after not eating for a while
- fatigue or tiredness
- unexplained weight loss
- unexplained iron deficiency in men, or in women after menopause

Treatment
- **Surgery** — This is the most common treatment. The affected malignant tumors and any nearby lymph nodes will be removed, to reduce the risk of the cancer spreading
- **Chemotherapy**
  - bevacizumab (Avastin)
  - ramucirumab (Cyramza)
- **Radiation therapy** — uses high energy radiation beams to destroy the cancer cells and to prevent them from multiplying
- **Ablation** — destroy a tumor without removing it; It can be carried out using radiofrequency, ethanol, or cryosurgery; These are delivered using a probe or needle that is guided by ultrasound or CT scanning technology

Risk factors
- older age
- diet that is high in animal protein, saturated fats, and calories
- diet that is low in fiber
- high alcohol consumption
- having bad breast, ovary, or uterine cancer
- having ulcerative colitis, Crohn's disease, or irritable bowel disease (IBD)
- The presence of polyps in the colon or rectum, as these may eventually become cancerous
- lack of physical activity
- overweight and obesity
- family history of colorectal cancer

Stages
- **Stage 0** — This is the earliest stage, when the cancer is still within the mucosa, or inner layer, of the colon or rectum
- **Stage 1** — The cancer has grown through the inner layer of the colon or rectum but has not yet spread beyond the wall of the rectum or colon
- **Stage 2** — The cancer has grown through or into the wall of the colon or rectum, but it has not yet reached the nearby lymph nodes
- **Stage 3** — The cancer has invaded the nearby lymph nodes, but it has not yet affected other parts of the body
- **Stage 4** — The cancer has spread to other parts of the body, including other organs, such as the liver, the membrane lining the abdominal cavity, the lung, or the ovaries
- **Recurrent** — The cancer has returned after treatment, it may come back and affect the rectum, colon, or another part of the body

Diagnosis
- **Fecal occult blood test (blood stool test)** — Blood may also be present because of other illnesses or conditions, such as hemorrhoids
- **Stool DNA test** — This test is more accurate for detecting colon cancer than polyps, but it cannot detect all DNA mutations that indicate that a tumor is present
- **Flexible sigmoidoscopy** — only detect polyps or cancer in the end third of the colon and the rectum
- **Barium enema X-ray** — Barium is a contrast dye that is placed into the patient's bowel in an enema form, and it shows up on an X-ray; the barium fills and coats the lining of the bowel, creating a clear image of the rectum, colon, and occasionally of a small part of the patient's small intestine
- **Colonoscopy** — It is a long, flexible, slender tube, attached to a video camera and monitor; The doctor can see the whole of the colon and rectum; Any polyps discovered during this exam can be removed during the procedure, and sometimes tissue samples, or biopsies, are taken instead
- **CT colonography** — A CT machine takes images of the colon, after closing the colon, if anything abnormal is detected, conventional colonoscopy may be necessary
- **Imaging scans** — Ultrasound or MRI scans can help show if the cancer has spread to another part of the body
- **Clinical tumor marker**
  - CA 19-9 (CEA)

Prevention
- **Regular screenings** — those who have had colorectal cancer before, who are over 50 years of age, who have a family history of this type of cancer, or have Crohn's disease should have regular screenings
- **Nutrition** — Follow a diet with plenty of fiber, fruit, vegetables, and good quality carbohydrates and a minimum of red and processed meats; Switch from saturated fats to good quality fats, such as avocado, olive oil, fish oils, and nuts
- **Exercise** — Moderate, regular exercise has been shown to have a significant impact on lowering a patient's risk of developing colorectal cancer
- **Bodyweight** — Being overweight or obese raises the risk of many cancers, including colorectal cancer

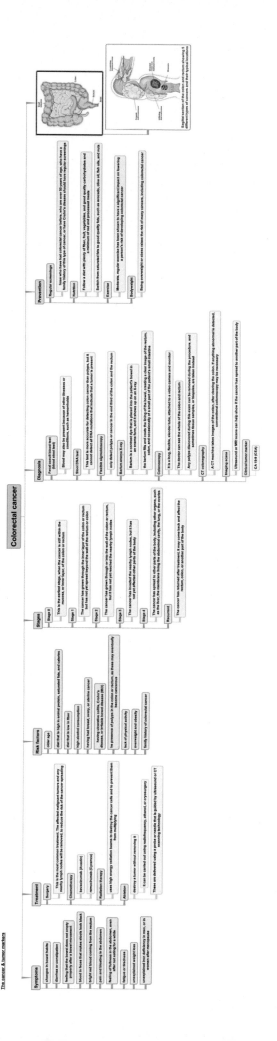

Sagittal section of the colon and rectum showing 5 different types of cancers and their typical locations

Kidney cancer

Symptoms
- blood in the urine
- lump or mass in the back, near the kidneys (one effect, three may be)
- a continuous pain in the side, near the kidneys
- anemia
- constant fever and night sweats
- tiredness or fatigue
- weight loss and loss of appetite

Treatment
- **Nephrectomy**
  - if the tumor is less than 1.5 inches, or 4 centimeters across, the surgeons may remove only part of the kidney in a partial nephrectomy
  - if the cancer has spread outside the kidney, surgery may not cure it, but it can ease pain and make other cancer-targeted treatments more effective
- **Embolization**
  - done to block the flow of blood to the tumor
  - the surgeon inserts a small tube known as a catheter into the groin
  - X-ray images guide the catheter into the blood supply for the kidney
  - A special material passed through the catheter into the blood vessel
  - blocking the blood supply to the kidney and starving the tumor of oxygen and nutrients
  - This causes the tumor to shrink
- **Cryoablation**
  - involves inserting one or more special needles, known as cryoprobes, through small incisions into the tumor
  - An imaging scan guides the process
  - A gas in the needles freezes the cells around the tip of each needle
  - Another gas warms these the cells, and then the cells are reheated
  - This freeze-thaw cycle kills the cancer cells
- **immunotherapy**
  - interferon
  - interleukin-2
- **is targeted therapy**
  - Axitinib, or Inlyta
  - Sorafenib, or Nexavar
  - Bevacizumab
  - Temsirolimus
- **Radiation therapy**
  - cannot usually cure kidney cancer, but it may help reduce the spread and the severity of symptoms

Stages
- **Stage 1**: The tumor is under 2.5 inches, or 7 centimeters in diameter and it is limited to the kidney
- **Stage 2**: The tumor is greater than 2.5 inches, or 7 centimeters, in diameter, and it is still limited to the kidney
- **Stage 3**: the tumor is any size but has spread beyond the kidney to at least one other location
  - the cancer may have reached the adrenal gland, nearby blood vessels, a lymph node, or the fat that surrounds the kidney
- **Stage 4**: the cancer has spread beyond the fatty tissue around the kidney, it affects at least one lymph node, or it has spread to other organs

Signs
- Blood and urine tests can rule out other possible causes of symptoms such as kidney stones or an infection
- ultrasound scan can help the doctor identify any change in the shape of the kidney that could be caused by a tumor
- CT scan normally involves the patient drinking a dye first
- Image-guided biopsy involves using a needle to remove a small sample of kidney tissue for examination under a microscope for cancer cells
- **Biopsy program**
  - A dye is injected into a vein in the patient's arm
  - The kidneys and urinary system process the dye, and this may enable any signs of cancer to show up on an X-ray
- **Cystoscopy**
  - A long narrow tube with a special lens and light at the end is inserted into the urethra, to provide an image inside the patient's bladder
  - A biopsy may be taken at the same time

Risk factors
- **Age**
  - This risk increases significantly after the age of 60 years
- **Sex**
  - For every two women who get kidney cancer, 3 men will do so
- **Obesity**
  - People with obesity have a significantly higher risk
- **Smoking**
  - Regular tobacco smokers have a much higher risk
  - but the risk drops when the person quits
- Workers who are exposed to chemicals
  - asbestos
  - cadmium
  - trichloroethylene
- Hypertension, or high blood pressure

Types
- urothelial cell carcinoma of the renal pelvis
- squamous cell carcinoma
- juxtaglomerular cell tumor, or reninoma
- angiomyolipoma
- renal oncocytoma
- Bellini duct carcinoma
- clear-cell adenoma of the kidney
- papillary nephroma
- Wilms' tumor, usually diagnosed in children under 5 years of age
- inherited kidney cancer caused by the loss or inactivation of a tumor suppressor gene called SFI on chromosome 11
- mixed epithelial stromal tumor

Prevention
- not smoking
- eating plenty of fruit and vegetables
- exercising regularly
- keeping the body weight within normal limits for your height, sex, and age
- getting at least 7 hours good quality continuous sleep every 24 hours
- maintaining a healthy blood pressure
- avoiding toxic chemicals

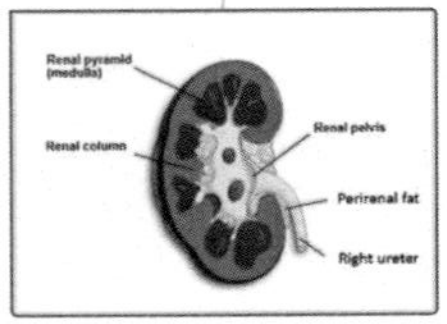

Kidney anatomy labels: Renal pyramid (medulla), Renal columns, Renal pelvis, Perirenal fat, Right ureter

The cancer & tumor markers

Lung Cancer

Symptoms
- Persistent or intense coughing
- Pain in the chest shoulder, or back from coughing
- Changes in color of the mucus that is coughed up from the lower airways (sputum)
- Difficulty breathing and swallowing
- Hoarseness of the voice
- Harsh sounds while breathing (stridor)
- Chronic bronchitis or pneumonia
- Coughing up blood, or blood in the sputum

Types of lung cancer
- Small cell lung cancer
  - Small cell lung cancer occurs almost exclusively in heavy smokers
  - less common than non-small cell lung cancer
- Non-small cell lung cancer
  - Include squamous cell carcinoma, adenocarcinoma and large cell carcinoma

stages
- Stage I
  - when the tumor is found only in one lung and in no lymph nodes
- Stage II
  - when the cancer has spread to the lymph nodes surrounding the infected lung
- Stage IIIa
  - when the cancer has spread to lymph nodes around the trachea, chest wall, and diaphragm, on the same side as the infected lung
- Stage IIIb
  - when the cancer has spread to lymph nodes on the other lung or in the neck
- Stage IV
  - when the cancer has spread throughout the rest of the body and other parts of the lungs.

Diagnosis
- Imaging tests
  - chest X-rays
  - CT scans
  - MRI scans
  - PET scans
  - bronchoscopy (a thin tube with a camera on one end)
- Sputum cytology
- Tissue sample (biopsy)
- Clinical tumor marker
  - CYFRA 21-1

Treatment
- Surgery
  - Procedures to remove lung cancer include
  - Wedge resection
    - to remove a small section of lung that contains the tumor along with a margin of healthy tissue
  - Segmental resection
    - to remove a larger portion of lung, but not an entire lobe
  - Lobectomy
    - to remove the entire lobe of one lung
  - Pneumonectomy
    - to remove an entire lung
- Radiation therapy
  - For people with locally advanced lung cancer, radiation may be used before surgery or after surgery
  - It's often combined with chemotherapy treatments
- Chemotherapy
  - used before surgery to shrink cancers and make them easier to remove
- Radiosurgery
  - Is an intense radiation treatment that aims many beams of radiation from many angles at the cancer
  - It may also be used to treat lung cancer that spreads to other parts of the body, including the brain
- Targeted drug therapy
  - focus on specific abnormalities present within cancer cells.
  - By blocking these abnormalities, targeted drug treatments can cause cancer cells to die
- Immunotherapy
- PARP (poly ADP ribose polymerase) inhibitors
  - 50% of PARP inhibitors could help treat patients with non-small-cell lung cancer

Risk factors
- Smoking
- Exposure to secondhand smoke
- Exposure to radon gas
- Exposure to asbestos and other carcinogens
- Family history of lung cancer

Prevention
- The most important preventive measure you can take to avoid lung cancer is to quit smoking.
- Eat a diet full of fruits and vegetables
- Exercise most days of the week

123

Melanoma

Symptoms
- **skin changes**
  - new spot or mole or a change in color, shape, or size of a current spot or mole
  - skin sore that fails to heal
  - spot or sore that becomes painful, itchy, or tender, or which bleeds
  - spot or lump that looks shiny, waxy, smooth, or pale
  - firm red lump that bleeds or appears ulcerated or crusty
  - flat, red spot that is rough, dry, or scaly

Stages
- **Stage 0**
  - melanoma in situ
  - The cancer is only in the outermost layer of skin
- **Stage 1**
  - The cancer is up to 2 millimeters (mm) thick
  - It has not spread to lymph nodes or other sites, and it may or may not be ulcerated
- **Stage 2**
  - The cancer is at least 1.01 mm thick and it may be thicker than 4 mm
  - It may or may not be ulcerated, and it has not yet spread to lymph nodes or other sites
- **Stage 3**
  - The cancer has spread to one or more lymph nodes or nearby lymphatic channels, but not to distant sites
  - The original cancer may no longer be visible. If it is visible, it may be thicker than 4 mm, and it may also be ulcerated
- **Stage 4**
  - The cancer has spread to distant lymph nodes or organs, such as the brain, lungs, or liver

Types
- **Superficial spreading melanoma**
  - appearing on the trunk or limbs
  - The cells tend to grow slowly at first, before spreading across the surface of the skin
- **Nodular melanoma**
  - appearing on the trunk, head, or neck
  - It tends to grow more quickly than other types, turning red—rather than black—as it grows
- **Lentigo maligna melanoma**
  - It starts as a Hutchinson's freckle, or lentigo maligna, which looks like a stain on the skin
  - It usually grows slowly and it less dangerous than other types
- **Acral lentiginous melanoma**
  - appearing on the palms of the hands, soles of the feet, or under the nails
  - It is more likely in people with darker skin and does not appear to be linked to sun exposure

Causes
- High freckle density or tendency to develop freckles after sun exposure
- presence of actinic lentigines, small gray-brown spots, also known as liver spots, sun spots, or age spots
- birth marks
- giant congenital melanocytic nevus, brown skin marks that present at birth
- pale skin that does not tan easily and burns, plus light-colored eyes
- red or light-colored hair
- high sun exposure
  - particularly if it produces blistering sunburn, and especially if sun exposure is intermittent rather than regular
- age, as risk increases with age
- family or personal history of melanoma
- having an organ transplant

ABCDE examination
- **Asymmetric**
  - normal moles are often round and symmetrical
  - whereas one side of a cancerous mole is likely to look different from the other side - not round or symmetrical
- **Border**
  - this is likely to be irregular rather than smooth - ragged, notched, or blurred
- **Color**
  - melanomas tend not to be of one color but to contain uneven shades and colors
  - including varying black, brown, and tan, and even white or blue pigmentation
- **Diameter**
  - a mole that is larger than a normal mole (more than a quarter inch in diameter) can indicate skin cancer
- **Evolving**
  - change in a mole's appearance over a period of weeks or months can be a sign of skin cancer

Diagnosis
- Physical examination of skin
- skin biopsy
  - Remove a sample of suspicious skin for testing

Treatment
- **Freezing**
  - destroy actinic keratoses and some small, early skin cancers by freezing them with liquid nitrogen (cryosurgery)
- **Excisional surgery**
  - cut out the cancerous tissue and a surrounding margin of healthy skin
- **Mohs surgery**
  - for larger, recurring, or difficult-to-treat skin cancers, which may include both basal and squamous cell carcinomas
- **Curettage and electrodesiccation or cryotherapy**
  - scrape away layers of cancer cells using a device with a circular blade (curet)
  - An electric needle destroys any remaining cancer cells
- liquid nitrogen can be used to freeze the base and edges of the treated area
- **Radiation therapy**
  - has cancer can't be completely removed during surgery
- **Chemotherapy**
- **Photodynamic therapy**
  - destroying skin cancer cells with a combination of laser light and drugs that makes cancer cells sensitive to light
- **Biological therapy**
  - using body's immune system to kill cancer cells

Prevention
- avoiding sunburn
- wearing clothes that protect against the sun
- using sunscreen with a minimum sun protection factor (SPF) of 15
  - but preferably SPF 20-30, with 4- or 5-star UVA protection
  - reapplying every 2 hours and after swimming to maintain adequate protection
- ❓ What about vitamin D?
  - Vitamin D is an important nutrient for the prevention of diseases such as rickets and osteomalacia
  - The time it takes to produce sufficient optimal vitamin D is less than the time it takes to get sunburnt
  - we can enjoy the sun safely and maintain optimal vitamin D levels without dramatically increasing the risk of skin cancer

124

The cancer & tumor markers

Spinal Cord Tumors

Symptoms

- Pain at the site of the tumor due to tumor growth
- Back pain, often radiating to other parts of your body
- Feeling less sensitive to pain, heat and cold
- Loss of bowel or bladder function
- Difficulty walking, sometimes leading to falls
- Back pain that's worse at night
- Loss of sensation or muscle weakness, especially in your arms or legs
- Muscle weakness, which may be mild or severe, in different parts of your body

classified into three major groups based on where they are found

- **Extradural Tumors**
  - Tumors between the bony spinal canal and the tough membrane called dura mater that protects the spinal cord
  - These are usually metastatic tumors and most often arise in the vertebrae themselves
- **(Intradural Tumors) Extramedullary Tumors**
  - Tumors inside the dura, but outside of spinal cord
  - These are usually nerve sheath tumors or meningiomas.
- **Intramedullary Tumors**
  - Tumors inside the spinal cord
  - These are usually astrocytomas or ependymomas

Treatment

- Monitoring
  - If small tumors aren't growing or pressing on surrounding tissues, watching them carefully may be all that's needed
- Surgery
- Radiation therapy
- Chemotherapy

Diagnosis

- Spinal magnetic resonance imaging (MRI)
- Computerized tomography (CT)
- Biopsy

Dura matter
Pia matter
Arachnoid matter
Spinal nerve
Transverse process
Vertebra
Intervertebral disc
Spinal cord

125

The cancer & tumor markers

COMMON CANCERS BY GENDER

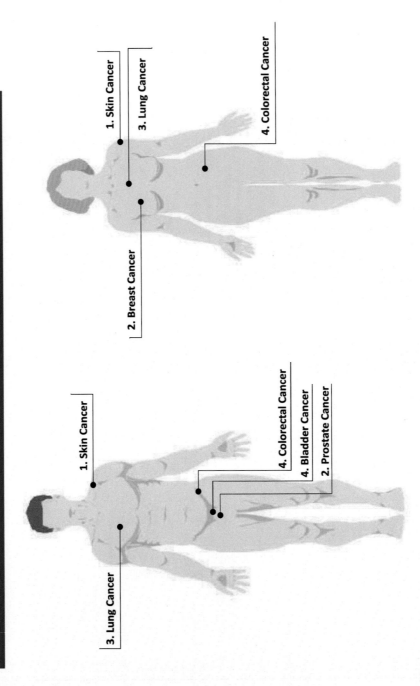

1. Skin Cancer
3. Lung Cancer
4. Colorectal Cancer
2. Breast Cancer

1. Skin Cancer
3. Lung Cancer
4. Colorectal Cancer
4. Bladder Cancer
2. Prostate Cancer

The cancer & tumor markers

Tumor marker is a bio marker found in blood, urine, or body tissues that can be elevated by the presence of one or more types of cancer

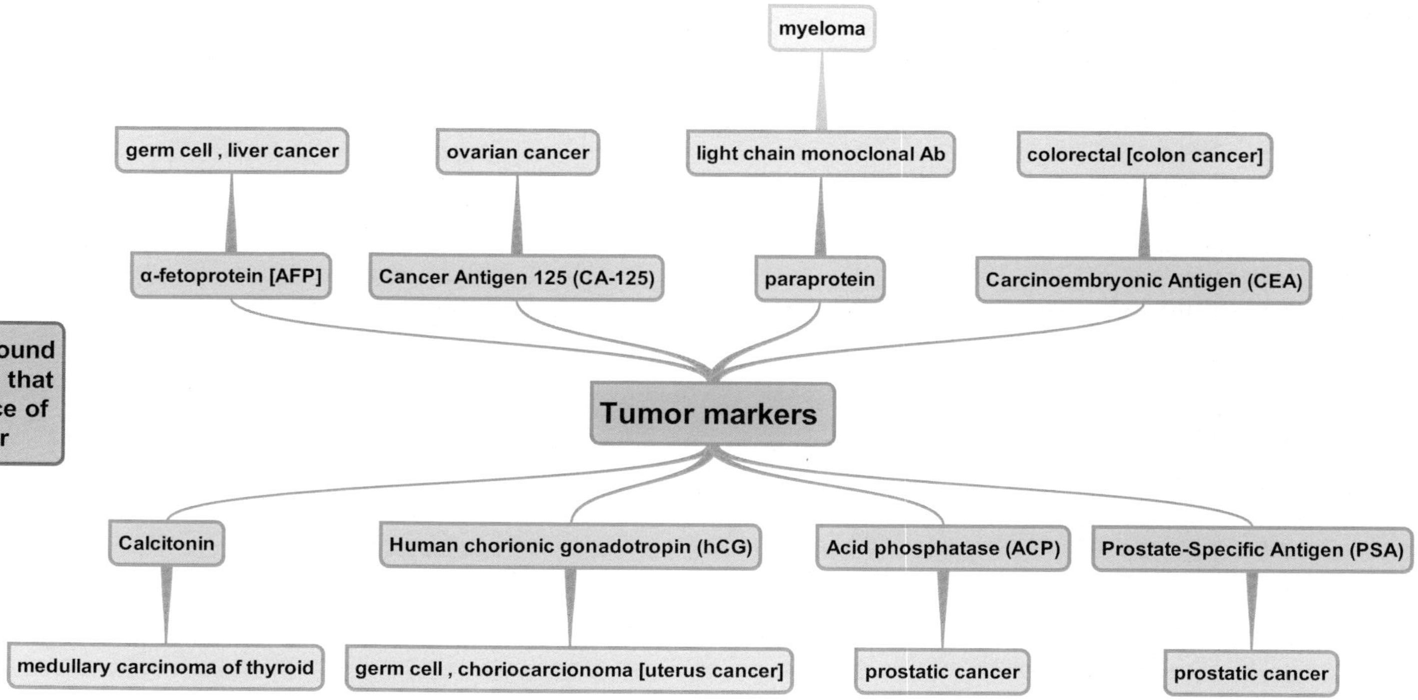

Tumor markers

- Carcinoembryonic Antigen (CEA)
  - colorectal [colon cancer]
- light chain monoclonal Ab
  - paraprotein — myeloma
- Cancer Antigen 125 (CA-125)
  - ovarian cancer
- α-fetoprotein [AFP]
  - germ cell , liver cancer
- Prostate-Specific Antigen (PSA)
  - prostatic cancer
- Acid phosphatase (ACP)
  - prostatic cancer
- Human chorionic gonadotropin (hCG)
  - germ cell , choriocarcionoma [uterus cancer]
- Calcitonin
  - medullary carcinoma of thyroid

127

The cancer & tumor markers

EXAMPLE OF TUMOR MARKERS

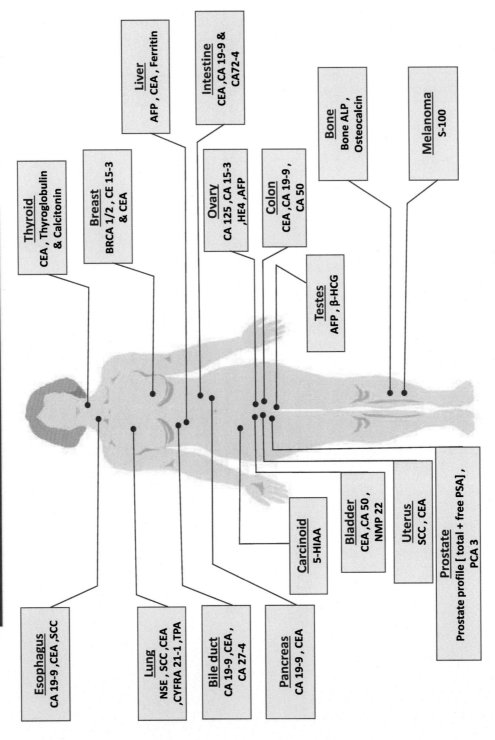

Esophagus
CA 19-9 ,CEA ,SCC

Thyroid
CEA , Thyroglobulin & Calcitonin

Breast
BRCA 1/2 , CE 15-3 & CEA

Liver
AFP , CEA , Ferritin

Intestine
CEA ,CA 19-9 & CA72-4

Lung
NSE , SCC ,CEA ,CYFRA 21-1 ,TPA

Ovary
CA 125 ,CA 15-3 ,HE4 ,AFP

Colon
CEA ,CA 19-9 , CA 50

Bone
Bone ALP , Osteocalcin

Melanoma
S-100

Bile duct
CA 19-9 ,CEA , CA 27-4

Testes
AFP , β-HCG

Pancreas
CA 19-9 , CEA

Carcinoid
5-HIAA

Bladder
CEA ,CA 50 , NMP 22

Uterus
SCC , CEA

Prostate
Prostate profile [total + free PSA] , PCA 3

128

Organ donation

you will organize your knowledge about :

Organs That Can Be Donated

- Heart
- Lung
- Liver
- Pancreas
- Kidney
- Intestine

Clinical Mind Maps
Biochemistry

129

Organs That Can Be Donated: Heart

Transplant Statistics

- Each year, about 2,000 heart transplants and fewer than 50 heart-lung transplants are performed

- In 2003, around 3,500 people were on the waiting list for a heart transplant and about 200 were waiting for a heart-lung transplant

- In 2003, over 450 people died while waiting for a heart transplant

- About 85 percent of heart transplant recipients are surviving one year after transplantation

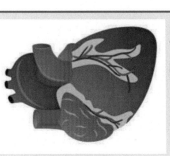

Diseases and Disorders

Cardiomyopathy
- is an abnormality of the heart muscle. The cause is often unknown.
- Advanced cases may require a heart transplant.

Myocarditis
- is an inflammation of the muscle tissue of the heart, often a complication of various infectious diseases.
- Severe cases can result in heart failure and require a heart transplant

Congestive Heart Failure
- is a condition resulting from heart disease such as coronary artery disease.
- The heart no longer pumps enough blood to meet the body's needs.
- A heart transplant may be needed if medical treatments fail

Congenital Heart Disease
- is the most common lethal birth defect, and the most common indication for heart transplantation in infants and young children

Organs That Can Be Donated: Intestine

Transplant Statistics

- Around 100 intestine transplants were performed in 2003

- In 2003, over 150 patients were on the waiting list for an intestine transplant

- In 2003, about 40 people died while waiting for an intestine transplant

- The one-year survival rate for intestine transplant recipients is about 60 percent

- The majority of intestinal transplants are performed in infants and children

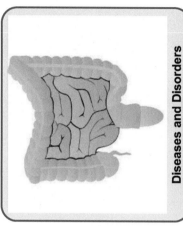

Diseases and Disorders

- Intestine transplants are required when the intestine becomes twisted and blocked or when there is irreversible intestinal failure.

- Most cases of intestinal failure are caused by short-gut syndrome (a significant loss of length of the small intestine present at birth or as a result of surgical removal or trauma).

- People with intestinal failure must receive nutrients intravenously.

- Because long-term intravenous feeding usually causes liver damage, many people who require a small intestine transplant also require a liver transplant at the same time.

Organs That Can Be Donated: Kidney

Transplant Statistics

About 14,000 kidney transplants are performed each year. Just over one third of transplanted kidneys are from living donors

At any point, about 55,000 people are on the waiting list for a kidney transplant

Every year, over 3,000 people die while waiting for a kidney transplant

The one-year survival rate for kidney transplant recipients is about 95 percent

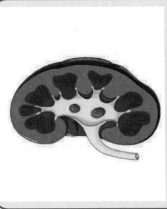

Diseases and Disorders

High blood pressure causes kidney damage, can lead to kidney failure, and is—as a result—an important predictor of kidney failure.

Diabetes is leading to kidney failure

People with severe kidney disease are often placed on dialysis machines

Other diseases (cystic kidney diseases) can cause the kidneys to become inflamed or can produce cysts in the kidneys that prevent them from functioning properly.

Organs That Can Be Donated: Liver

Transplant Statistics

Around 5,000 people receive liver transplants each year

Each year, over 17,000 people are waiting to receive a liver transplant

Each year, about 2,000 people die while waiting for a liver

One year after the surgery, about 85 percent of liver transplant recipients live fairly normal lives

A donated liver can be split between two recipients, so that one deceased donor can be the source of two liver transplants

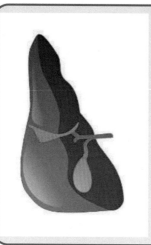

Diseases and Disorders

Damage from alcohol and other drugs. Damage from blood clots in the liver

Chronic liver infections, such as hepatitis (particularly B and C), which severely damage the liver

Birth defects of the liver or bile duct

The skin of people with liver damage may turn yellow from a condition called jaundice.

They also may gain weight and experience general weakness.

Because the liver is involved in many metabolic processes, severe liver damage is often fatal.

Organs That Can Be Donated: Lung

Transplant Statistics

- About 1,000 patients receive a lung transplant each year
- Each year, about 4,000 people are waiting for a lung transplant
- Over 400 people die each year while waiting for a lung transplant
- About 75 percent of lung transplant recipients survive the first year
- A single lung can save a life. One deceased donor can be the source of two lung transplants

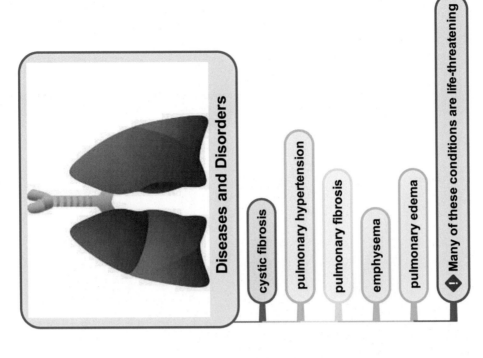

Diseases and Disorders

- cystic fibrosis
- pulmonary hypertension
- pulmonary fibrosis
- emphysema
- pulmonary edema
- ❗ Many of these conditions are life-threatening

Organs That Can Be Donated: Pancreas

Transplant Statistics

In 2003, over 450 people received a pancreas transplan

In 2003, about 1,500 people were on the waiting list for a pancreas

In 2003, about 30 people died while waiting for a pancreas transplant

One year after receiving a pancreas transplant, about 95 percent of recipients are still living

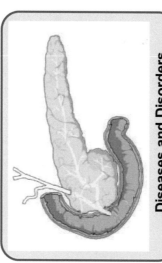

Diseases and Disorders

Malfunction or failure of the pancreas leads to diabetes—an inability to control the level of glucose in the blood

Individuals with this condition are called diabetics and may need insulin to control the level of glucose in the blood.

Diabetes can damage or cause the failure of many of the body's organs

Because patients requiring a pancreas transplant often have kidney disease, the pancreas and kidneys are sometimes transplanted together.

Failure to treat diabetes can lead to organ failure and death.

protein misfolding diseases

you will organize your knowledge about :

The symptoms, diagnosis, and treatment for degenerative diseases

Alzheimer's disease

Parkinson's disease

protein misfolding diseases

Alzheimer's Disease

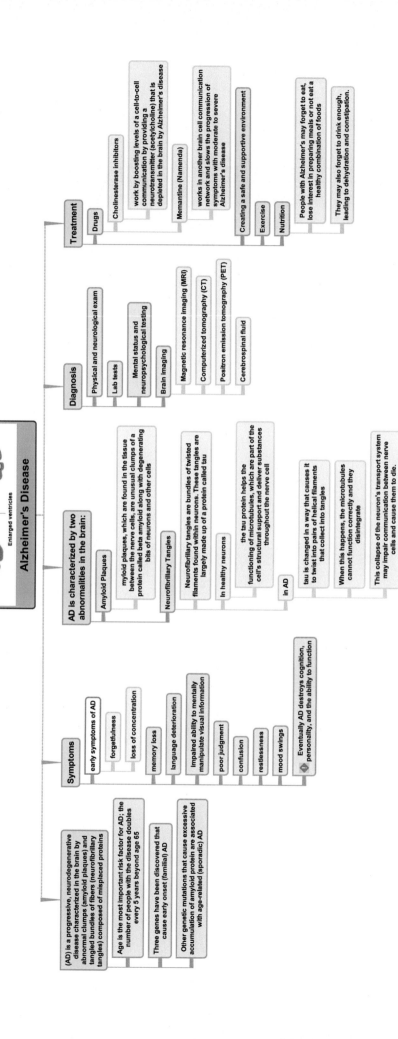

Shrinkage of cerebral cortex

Enlarged ventricles

(AD) is a progressive, neurodegenerative disease characterized in the brain by abnormal clumps (amyloid plaques) and tangled bundles of fibers (neurofibrillary tangles) composed of misplaced proteins

Age is the most important risk factor for AD; the number of people with the disease doubles every 5 years beyond age 65

Three genes have been discovered that cause early onset (familial) AD

Other genetic mutations that cause excessive accumulation of amyloid protein are associated with age-related (sporadic) AD

Symptoms

early symptoms of AD
- forgetfulness
- loss of concentration

memory loss

language deterioration

Impaired ability to mentally manipulate visual information

poor judgment

confusion

restlessness

mood swings

Eventually AD destroys cognition, personality, and the ability to function

AD is characterized by two abnormalities in the brain:

Amyloid Plaques

myloid plaques, which are found in the tissue between the nerve cells, are unusual clumps of a protein called beta amyloid along with degenerating bits of neurons and other cells

Neurofibrillary Tangles

Neurofibrillary tangles are bundles of twisted filaments found within neurons. These tangles are largely made up of a protein called tau

In healthy neurons

the tau protein helps the functioning of microtubules, which are part of the cell's structural support and deliver substances throughout the nerve cell

in AD

tau is changed in a way that causes it to twist into pairs of helical filaments that collect into tangles

When this happens, the microtubules cannot function correctly and they disintegrate

This collapse of the neuron's transport system may impair communication between nerve cells and cause them to die.

Diagnosis

Physical and neurological exam

Lab tests

Mental status and neuropsychological testing

Brain imaging
- Magnetic resonance imaging (MRI)
- Computerized tomography (CT)
- Positron emission tomography (PET)

Cerebrospinal fluid

Treatment

Drugs

Cholinesterase inhibitors

work by boosting levels of a cell-to-cell communication by providing a neurotransmitter (acetylcholine) that is depleted in the brain by Alzheimer's disease

Memantine (Namenda)

works in another brain cell communication network and slows the progression of symptoms with moderate to severe Alzheimer's disease

Creating a safe and supportive environment

Exercise

Nutrition

People with Alzheimer's may forget to eat, lose interest in preparing meals or not eat a healthy combination of foods

They may also forget to drink enough, leading to dehydration and constipation.

137

<u>Protein misfolding diseases</u>

Parkinson's Disease

symptoms

(PD) is a neurodegenerative disorder of the central nervous system

movement disorders

- tremor
  - trembling in hands, arms, legs, jaw, or head
- rigidity, or stiffness of the limbs and trunk
- bradykinesia, or slowness of movement
- postural instability, or impaired balance
- symptoms usually begin gradually and worsen with time

Caudate nucleus
Putamen
Striatum
Substantia nigra
Thalamus
Cerebellum

Diagnosis

- dopamine transporter (DAT) scan
  - specific single-photon emission computerized tomography SPECT scan
- lab tests, such as blood tests
- Imaging tests — such as MRI, CT, ultrasound of the brain, and PET scans
- Parkinson's disease medication
  - carbidopa-levodopa (Rytary, Sinemet, others)

Treatment

- Medications
  - Carbidopa-levodopa
    - Levodopa is combined with carbidopa (Lodosyn)
      - which protects levodopa from early conversion to dopamine outside your brain
      - This prevents or lessens side effects such as nausea.
  - Carbidopa-levodopa infusion
  - Dopamine agonists
  - MAO B inhibitors
  - Catechol O-methyltransferase (COMT) inhibitors
  - Anticholinergics
  - Amantadine
- Surgical procedures
  - Deep brain stimulation
    - surgeons implant electrodes into a specific part of brain
    - electrodes are connected to a generator implanted in chest near collarbone
    - that sends electrical pulses to your brain and may reduce Parkinson's disease symptoms
    - it doesn't keep Parkinson's disease from progressing

138

References

1. Allan Gaw; Michael J. Murphy; Robert A. Cowan; Denis St. J. O`Reilly; Michael J. Stewart; James Shepherd. Clinical biochemistry. 4th edition. CHURCHIL LIVINGSTONE: ELSEVIER. 2008.

2. Amitava Dasgupta. Alcohol and its Biomarkers. Clinical Aspects and Laboratory Determination. 2015

3. Attallah AM, El-Far M, Abdallah SO, El-Waseef AM, Omran MM, Abdelrazek MA, Attallah AA, Saadh MJ, Radwan M, El-waffaey KA, Abol-Enei H. Combined use of epithelial membrane antigen and nuclear matrix protein 52 as sensitive biomarkers for detection of bladder cancer. Int J Biol Markers. 11;30(4). 2015. Robert L. Sunheimer; Linda Grave. Clinical Laboratory Chemistry. 1st edition. 2010.

4. Carl A. Burtis; David E. Bruns. Tietz Fundamentals of Clinical Chemistry and Molecular Diagnostics (Fundamentals of Clinical Chemistry (Tietz)). 7th edition. 2014.

5. Martin A. Crook. Clinical chemistry and metabolic medicine. 7th edition. BookPower. 2006

6. Mayoclinic. https://www.mayoclinic.org/departments-centers

7. Medical news today. https://www.medicalnewstoday.com/

8. Michael L. Bishop; Edward P. Fody; Laary E. Shoff. Clinical Chemistry: Principles, Techniques, and Correlations.8th edition. 2017.

9. William J. Marshall; Stephen K. Bangert; Marta Lapsley. Clinical chemistry. 7th edition. MOSBY: ELSEVIER. 2012.

Mind Maps

Clinical Biochemistry

Printed in the United States
By Bookmasters